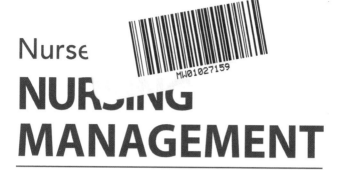

Nurse

NURSING
MANAGEMENT

FOLLOW THESE INSTRUCTIONS
TO DOWNLOAD:

1) Use your Web browser to go to:
   http://www.mhnursetonurse.com

2) Register now

3) Fill in the required fields

4) Enter your unique registration code below

5) Download the software and sync into your
   handheld device

Code Listed Here

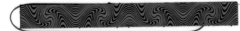

**NOTE: BOOK IS NOT RETURNABLE ONCE
SCRATCH-OFF IS REMOVED**

Scratch off coating above to reveal your unique code
to download your mobile device software.

See above for complete directions.

If you have any problems accessing your download,
please email: techsolutions@mhedu.com

P/N 9780071601559
0071601554
part of set
ISBN 978-0-07-160153-5
MHID 0-07-160153-8

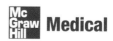

mcgraw-hillmedical.com

Nurse to Nurse
NURSING MANAGEMENT

Nurse to Nurse
NURSING
MANAGEMENT

Linda J. Knodel, MHA, MSN, RN, CPHQ, NE-BC, FACHE
Senior Vice President/Chief Nursing Officer
St. Alexius Medical Center
Bismarck, North Dakota

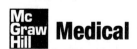 **Medical**

New York Chicago San Francisco Lisbon London Madrid Mexico City
Milan New Delhi San Juan Seoul Singapore Sydney Toronto

The **McGraw·Hill** Companies

Nurse to Nurse: Nursing Management

1 2 3 4 5 6 7 8 9 0   DOC/DOC   14 13 12 11 10 9

Set 978-0-07-160153-5 MHID: 0-07-160153-8
Book 978-0-07-160154-2 MHID: 0-07-160154-6
Card 978-0-07-160155-9 MHID: 0-07-160155-4

This book was set in Berkeley Book by Glyph International.
The editors were Joseph Morita and Karen Davis.
The production supervisor was Catherine H. Saggese.
Production management was provided by Ekta Dixit, Glyph International.
The book designer was Eve Siegel.
The cover designer was David Dell'Accio.
The index was prepared by Robert Swanson.
RR Donnelley was printer and binder.

This book is printed on acid-free paper.

Library of Congress Cataloging-in-Publication Data

Knodel, Linda J.
    Nurse to nurse : nursing management / Linda J. Knodel.
        p. ; cm.
    Includes bibliographical references and index.
    ISBN-13: 978-0-07-160153-5 (pbk. : alk. paper)
    ISBN-10: 0-07-160153-8 (alk. paper)
    1. Nursing services—Administration.   2. Nurse administrators.
I. Title.
    [DNLM: 1. Nursing, Supervisory.   2. Clinical Competence.
3. Education, Nursing.   4. Leadership.   5. Nursing Care—organization &
administration.   6. Nursing Care—standards.   WY 105 K72n 2010]
    RT89.K66 2010
    362.17'3068—dc22
                             2009036596

Contents

Preface

Two thousand nine has been a year of extraordinary change in the United States: We have witnessed a history-making new president, unprecedented economic concerns, escalating environmental threats, and significant shifts in corporate accountability. Although it feels as if most of the world is experiencing a "perfect storm" of uncertainty and chaos, this type of turbulence is actually familiar within health care.

I am a chief nursing officer. I have been a nurse for over 30 years, and in my career I have seen amazing changes in the people and the processes for delivering care. As part of my role, I also am involved with numerous health care societies on the regional and national level. As I talk with my colleagues throughout the nation, it is obvious that the pace of change is ebbing and flowing in intensity . . . with a pretty significant increase upon us now.

The world of nursing has seen some of the most profound changes in the past 50 years. The advent of clinical, informational, and personal technology as well as shifts in revenue sources and expense management, documentation and reporting programs, and programs focusing on patient safety and quality have taken nursing to a place we never could have imagined in the 1960s.

Along with those evolutions (or should I say, revolutions?), we also have witnessed a changing workforce. Today's nurses are older, come from different nations and walks of life, and have different levels of training. By 2020, the United States will need far more nurses than will be available. Although we are working to educate nurses as quickly as possible, we also need to equip them with the skills and resiliency to weather the changes still to come.

I am convinced that the key to our future is leadership, and that is why I wrote this book. The entire nursing workforce is aging. Those who have been leaders are approaching retirement. More than that threat, however, we must recognize that the role of leaders (and the preparation for leadership) is also changing.

In addition to the common issues confronting nursing as a profession, diverse issues exist that are unique to each community, state, and region. I therefore felt it imperative that the initial manuscript proposal for this book incorporate feedback from key nurse leaders across the nation. I asked these leaders the following questions:

1. What keeps you awake at night?
2. What five things give you nightmares?
3. What will we be judged on over the next 10 years?
4. What standards are front-line managers being required to meet?
5. What are the top 10 issues or guiding principles?
6. What are the burning issues for aspiring nurse leaders?
7. How do you accurately coach an individual so that he or she will not burn out?
8. What has been your greatest success in the past 3 years—the one that made a difference and garnered recognition for your organization?
9. Is there a particular story you would like to share as it relates to any of the aforementioned issues?

Since the days of Florence Nightingale, the nurse has always been the navigator of patient care. Nurses are recognized for their knowledge and caring, the essence of what they bring to the health care field. It is essential that these aspects never be lost, and that they be enhanced significantly through nursing leadership reform. Such reform is necessary not only to deal with the ongoing changes that are occurring at warp speed today, but also to encourage the thought leaders of tomorrow.

The driving forces that keep nursing executives awake at night are the financial woes of the health care system. Single-handedly, finances drive the entire spectrum of health care. We regularly hear, "No margin, no mission." As leaders we also recognize the greatest financial appropriation within a health care system is the nursing staff.

Regulation continues to increase, and continuous reporting demands abound. The resources necessary to accomplish this task often come at the expense of the bedside caregiver—the nurse— who often is responsible for ensuring that such imperatives are met, without having additional resources to assist in the process. The mantra of nursing, "Add, add, add, and never take away," is a reality.

The nursing shortage that continues to loom affects not only bedside caregivers but also the faculty needed to prepare them for the role. At the same time, today's states are passing legislation to promote increased enrollment in nursing schools.

An enormous void exists between governance and executives who do not understand the business of patient care. Emphasis on technology continues to be at the forefront; however, few organizations are able to afford the expense associated with it. Therefore, care is provided with great variability while at the same time the expectations by consumers and payers for quality outcomes abound.

As nurse leaders of today, we will be judged on the basis of our role in upholding patient safety, our creativity in providing the necessary resources for the bedside nurse, and our advocacy of baccalaureate education as the minimum preparation for a nursing career. This is based on the "critical synthesis" that will be required to carry out the work of the nurse of the future. It behooves nurse leaders to be present and to ensure that our voices are heard where national policy is made.

Academia plays a significant role in influencing teamwork among health care providers. Programs continue to be taught in "silos"; it is no wonder that care is provided accordingly. When will the nation recognize the need for governance, leadership, and providers to gather as thought leaders and develop delivery models that will guide us efficiently and effectively into the future?

If the United States is unable to provide the necessary nursing resources, introducing foreign-trained staff will require additional educational and leadership competencies. As less-invasive technology is introduced (and becomes an expectation of the consumer), our ability to respond to complex patient care needs in a far shorter period of time must also be addressed.

Far too often, the voice of the nurse is forgotten amid the need to have the best MRI scanner or robot. Yes, the use of less-invasive procedures decreases the time spent in the hospital, yet the issues surrounding the patient care plan do not decrease. How, then, can nurses collaborate with the rest of the health care team as well as the payers within health care?

Future nurse leaders must recognize that change is constant and they must have the ability to deal with ambiguity. Having a voice at the executive "table" as an equal partner to finance is imperative. Nursing can break or make a system; without nursing, the need to worry about finances will be nonexistent.

These and numerous other principles must be core elements in any curriculum for leadership. No longer can we assume that just because someone is an excellent clinical nurse, that person will be an excellent nurse leader. The nursing profession is responsible not only for recognizing the various roles but also for providing the education and training necessary for nurses to do their jobs to meet our needs of the future.

This book not only addresses controversial issues surrounding health care, but also provides a pathway to enhance the health care system. Nursing alone does not hold all the answers because providing care is a team effort whose many stakeholders influence the work of the nurse. To understand the dynamics involved and develop the future state in which health care leadership will operate, one must understand the current state. Nursing is central to the health care team. As leaders, we owe it to the profession today as well as to nurses of the future to develop this guide.

This book can and will be used in undergraduate and graduate curricula for all of the health care professions. Its applicability to the health care setting ensures that the book will assist current and future nurse leaders to grow even further.

Contained in this book are exercises that can be used by multidisciplinary teams to assess the effectiveness of their roles and identify whether areas for improvement or options for change exist. The book also provides current and future nurse leaders with tools to assist them in the continuous development of leadership teams as well as succession planning.

This book has the potential to assist the entire health care team as the essential leadership handbook. It is designed to help those who aspire to be nurse leaders, as well as existing leaders and nursing faculty. It is a high-level resource, a primer of sorts, describing the key elements of nursing leadership.

By no means is this book exhaustive. It does, however, respond to the important questions and issues that have influenced my own work and that of my colleagues. I wrote this book to begin a conversation that I hope nurses and their mentors will continue to have throughout the nation. Luckily, I am not alone in this idea. Quoted in *Modern Healthcare* on March 23, 2009, President Obama described the need to support nursing education and development by saying, "There are a lot of people (in the United States) who would love to be in that helping profession, and yet we just aren't providing the resources to get them trained—that's something that we've got to fix. That should be a no-brainer."* I couldn't agree more, and so I invite you to participate in this dialogue with me.

Special acknowledgment goes to my colleagues who assisted me in this effort from St. Alexius Medical Center, Bismarck, North Dakota:

- Andrew L. Wilson, President/CEO
- Gary P. Miller, CPA, Senior Vice President/Chief Financial Officer
- Tim Blasl, Patient Financial Services and Reimbursement Director
- Frank Kilzer, Vice President of Material and Facility Resources
- Karen A. Schneider, MS, RN, NP, CNN, Director, Regional Renal Services & Apheresis

---

*Some support visas for nurses; Obama doesn't. *Modern Healthcare*, March 23, 2009. Available at: http://www.modernhealthcare.com/apps/pbcs.dll/article?AID=/20090323/SUB/903209972/1139&nocache=1.

- Donna Gage, MMgmt, NE-BC, Director of Emergency/Trauma, Medical, Surgical, & Oncology Units
- Jody Benz, MSN, NE-BC, Director, Women's and Children's Units
- Victoria Thomas, Executive Assistant, Administration
- Pamela Kling, Executive Assistant, Administration
- Jenni Yoder, Nursing Secretary, Nursing Services

Linda J. Knodel, MHA, MSN, RN, CPHQ, NE-BC, FACHE
Senior Vice President/Chief Nursing Officer
St. Alexius Medical Center
Bismarck, North Dakota
September 2009

Acknowledgments

Aside from the individuals whose contributions to health care, nursing leadership, academia and public policy assisted me in the development of this book, a note of special recognition is owed to Ms. Virginia Tyler, Rochester, New York. Without your time, talent, and guidance, this book would not have been possible. I am grateful for our friendship, long discussions and your ongoing encouragement.

In reflecting about the numerous individuals who provided the early molding necessary to write this book, I would like to note that my mother Anne Redman Carns, a school teacher, and my father William Carns, a business owner, provided the environment in my formative years that encouraged diversity and always allowed for ongoing personal growth. The Benedictine Sisters of the Annunciation Monastery, Bismarck North Dakota, provided the values based professional laboratory for me to practice and at the same time continuously grow and influence others along the way.

Honoring my family is the greatest testimony of all to this book. Each member of my family will notably recall the vacations which were spent writing. My husband, Ken Albert Knodel, creatively found activities with family and friends so that I could have quiet time to write. You are my hero! I would also like to acknowledge my three wonderful daughters and son-in-law Kristen B. Knodel, MD; Kendra Leigh Knodel, RN, WHNP; Katie (Knodel) Kummer, MA, MS and Andrew Kummer, MD for your encouragement, inspiration, and real life examples for my very first book. You are the greatest support a mother, wife and nurse leader could ever dream of.

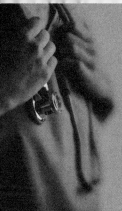

Chapter 1

OVERVIEW OF NURSING LEADERSHIP

"Nursing management is as much a nursing specialty as any specialty and requires specialty leadership skills. Mentorship/leadership from senior leaders smoothes the transition from clinical roles to formal leadership roles. At the same time, nurse leaders must learn the business side of healthcare while maintaining the care side"

—Kathleen Sanford, DBA, RN, FACHE;
Senior Vice President, Chief Nursing Officer,
Catholic Health Initiatives,
Denver, Colorado

WHAT IS LEADERSHIP?

Let's begin by defining leadership. There are many different competencies within the field of leadership but generally speaking, leadership is the ability to define a vision and guide individuals and groups toward that vision while maintaining group-promoting teamwork, commitment, and effectiveness. Teamwork embraces the productive aspects of group cohesion and it focuses on the leader's ability to ensure that team member relationships are collaborative and productive.

Guiding assists those being guided to "connect the dots." Leadership provides the foundation for motivation and sets the stage for obtaining commitment, rather than merely compliance, from those being guided. Guiding does not become the end point—it is part of the execution that leads to individual awareness, which sets the stage for behavioral change.

Leadership has been (and continues to be) one of the most studied and written-about topics. Going back more than 2000 years, even the great philosopher Confucius wrote about the elements of good leadership. He noted that domineering styles of management, based on top-down principles, were not as successful as creating a structure based on rules. In other words, people respond better when they know both why something is important and what the guidelines are to achieving the organization's outcome. Confucius also recognized that "leading by example" was important to strong leadership, as well as honing virtues such as respect and humility.

In my years of working alongside other nurse leaders and serving as faculty for the American Organization of Nurse Executives' Aspiring Nurse Leaders Institute, I have often observed that when people think about leadership, they tend to think about the characteristics of the person and not necessarily the tactical elements of the person's job. If I ask aspiring leaders to close their eyes and reflect on the leader they most admire, invariably they will describe that leader as honest, caring, supportive, guiding, teaching, and kind.

What they tend not to describe is how the leader does the job. They do not say that a good leader never misses a day of work, or that good leaders are wizards at finance, able to develop programs that save their departments lots of money. Neither do they say that good leaders are doctorally prepared nor that they receive awards. They do not describe how many meetings the leader attends, or how the leader dresses. Instead, they describe who the leaders are as people. Their responses seem to mirror the new yardstick and measurement model developed by Daniel Goleman in his 1998 book, *Working with Emotional Intelligence*.[1] Goleman highlights four main points in his model:

1. Self-awareness, defined as the ability to read one's emotions and recognize their impact while using instinct to guide decisions.
2. Self-management, which involves mastering one's emotions and impulses and adapting to changing circumstances.
3. Social awareness, the ability to sense, understand, and react to others' emotions while comprehending the networks by which people interact.
4. Relationship management, which involves inspiring, influencing, and developing others while managing conflict.

The above domains describe how a leader handles himself or herself as well as how she or he works with others. Goleman notes that these acquired skills and competencies predict positive outcomes, whether at work, with family, or with friends.

It should be noted that very few students point to leadership in their academic field as being a career goal. They do not say they want to be the dean of a college, for example, although they may say that they aspire to be the president of a company, a chief executive officer, a chairman of the board of directors, a principal, a governor, and so on.

In fact, when we think about leadership in narrow terms, as referring only to being the ultimate person in charge of an organization or system, we overlook the many leadership positions that exist at various levels and times throughout life. Further, when we take on leadership positions, it is often a result of specific factors and timing, and our instinct to step up is based on a desire to help rather than a need to be in charge.

IMPRESSIONS OF LEADERSHIP

We should acknowledge that leadership opportunities are available throughout our work and professional lives—not simply the point at which we finish a degree or achieve a particular level of certification. For example, children have opportunities to become leaders when they are named the captain of a sports team or the president of a scout troop or dance club. Their leadership role as captain or club officer provides them with additional responsibilities and opportunities for learning. These early exposures to leadership are great testing points for young people. Over the course of their leadership experience, they can determine whether this type of role—with its added responsibility, visibility, and work—is something they want to pursue in the future.

Young people are often exposed to leadership through their families. By observing their parents, siblings, and other relatives in their work and community life, they may see opportunities to influence their community and create a positive place to live. However, along with the benefits of having a leader in their midst, family members sometimes experience the difficulties that accompany leadership. Children may find that their leader-parent is not available as much as they might like because of other commitments. When a parent is not available for homework help, or misses a school event, it may create confusion or a bad impression that stays with the child for years afterward.

Similar impressions of a leadership role can develop in the work setting. Within a work group, staff members may observe the long hours that their leader puts in without understanding the various tasks and responsibilities that she or he faces each day. Staff persons may observe that unlike their own shifts, which are completed in 8 hours, their leader's "shift" goes on and on, as he or she takes work home on weekends and during the week. This, too, creates an impression of the role of leadership. The observing employee may view the leader as being overwhelmed with work or infer that the person is not able to prioritize. However, often the need for extended hours and additional work is based on other factors entirely.

For example, to facilitate communication with trauma surgeons and the trauma team, the best time to meet may be at 6 AM. Community and board meetings may need to take place in the evenings to facilitate the work schedules of attendees. Leaders understand that their role is not defined by an 8-hour workday and that adapting to the schedule is simply part of their position. Variability and flexibility are important elements for leaders to embrace. Likewise, good leaders will communicate and provide a context for their peers to help them understand why schedules and workloads appear as they do.

Continuing with the preceding example, most organizations have a board of directors. Their role is to represent the interests of the community while also providing advice and counsel to the organization. The members of the board are leaders themselves, and their input into the organization is vital. The diversity of their thinking is crucial to the organization's success because they take management thinking outside the organization's internal vacuum and provide a different perspective. Their outside input assists in making the business more effective and successful. The cross-pollination of learning among leaders, as well as their different styles and perspectives, gives even greater support and intelligence to organizational decision making. It also promotes greater leadership growth for all of the participants.

In most cases, these board members are volunteers. Staff leaders working with the board understand that, as part of their own leadership role, they must meet with and receive information from the board through meetings that are not interrupted by the day-to-day work of the organization. For both the volunteer leader and the staff leader, these meetings occur outside of working hours; thus, involvement becomes a personal decision and commitment. How leaders present the value of this added responsibility is vitally important. Choosing to participate in an organization's leadership group (whether as a volunteer or as a staff person) will have both a short-term and a long-term impact on the community in which the organization operates. Family members, staff members, and colleagues can be encouraged to view the leader's involvement as a valuable commitment to improving lives rather than as time away from home or work life.

Leadership is a feature not only of our own organizations, but of our industries as well. In health care, serving at the local, regional, or national level provides a great vantage point from the field and a network second to none. One can read the literature again and again; however, exposure to the field provides an even greater opportunity for personal and organizational growth.

For the purpose of this discussion, the focus in the rest of this chapter will be on choice—specifically, choosing leadership as a career path. This choice, as noted above, can and will have implications. What these implications will be depends in large part on the frame that is placed around these choices, and on the individual's attitude and ability to articulate the impact leadership has on his or her personal and professional life.

WHO BECOMES A NURSE LEADER, AND HOW?

People who become nurse leaders tend to have two qualities. First and foremost, they are excellent clinicians. Often, they also have innate leadership acumen, meaning they are natural mentors and informal opinion guides for their peers. These are the nurses that younger nurses seek out for clinical, professional, and even personal advice. They are also the nurses most likely to identify opportunities for improvement and volunteer to lead the improvement initiative.

Simply because a nurse has clinical expertise and acumen does not mean he or she will be immediately successful as a leader. Once tapped by management to assume an entry-level leadership position, new leaders often struggle with how to transfer their informal leadership capability into the formal role. Both the individual leader and his or her peers experience a change as the new leader is separated out by title and responsibility. Without some formalized means to learn their new role, many new leaders become frustrated. They want to succeed in the position, but the adjustment can be difficult when those who were "stars" before assuming the formalized leadership role are not immediately stars in the new role. In such cases, frustration and misaligned expectations often lead to a new leader's failure.

Many organizations try to help young leaders by providing a mentor. Mentorship can help in the short run by providing a trusted guide to the operational aspects of the new role. However, mentorship runs the risk of creating many different types of leaders as each mentee adopts the style and the approach of the respective mentor. Such emulation is to be expected: Every learner mirrors and repeats the beliefs, processes, and opinions of the teacher. Over time, however, the organization risks creating multiple "right approaches" based on differing styles of the individual mentors. As we will discuss at length in chapter 3, variation is one of the greatest dangers in health care. The same is true in training new leaders. Without a standardized process for identifying, training, and supporting leaders (at every level), an organization risks significant variation in how leaders lead. We will discuss these issues further in chapters 6 and 7.

In the meantime, nurse leaders continue to emerge from the pool of strong clinicians who have stable and abiding relationships with their organizations. For individuals who aspire to leadership roles, there is always value in shadowing leaders; participating in councils, committees, and task forces; and studying the formal and informal roles that leaders hold.

WHO ARE THE LEADERS IN HEALTH CARE ORGANIZATIONS, AND WHAT ARE THE TOOLS THEY USE IN LEADING?

For the purpose of this discussion, we will limit our focus to hospitals, because the majority of nurses work in hospital settings. Hospitals have numerous types and levels of leaders, all working together.

The highest authority within a hospital is the board of directors (also known as the governing body). The board is a group of individuals who, by virtue of their community role, health care expertise, business acumen, and interest, are appointed for terms typically ranging between 2 and 4 years. Most often, board members are volunteers, although certain members of the board, such as the hospital chief executive officer, chief financial officer, chief medical officer (and in some cases chief nursing officer), may sit on the board *ex officio*, which means "by virtue of their office." *Ex officio* members may or may not have voting privileges on the board. The board is responsible for all activities of the hospital, including finances, quality, service configuration, medical staff appointments, and employee performance. The hospital board is ultimately responsible for ensuring that safe and appropriate care is provided to the community. It is accountable to patients, the general public, payers, and the government. About 18% of community hospitals are investor-owned for-profit businesses.[2] In those cases, the board is also responsible to the organization's investors.

All boards use a set of rules (or bylaws) to guide their actions. The bylaws specify everything from how often the board meets, to how many seats it has, to the role and process of board-level committees, including, for example, the finance committee, audit committee, credentialing committee, quality committee, strategic planning committee, and others. No two boards operate exactly alike; therefore, the bylaws are an important tool used in the board's work.

The board or governing body sets the direction for the organization. Management, in turn, is responsible for implementing the direction established by the governing body. Examples of such direction may include

1. The mission to be achieved or sustained by the organization will be defined.
2. Employee satisfaction will meet or exceed benchmark.
3. The net bottom line will achieve a certain percentage.
4. Average age of plant will not exceed a certain age.
5. Quality ratings will be within a certain percentile of all hospitals reporting.

6. Capital expenditure will not exceed a certain dollar amount without express board approval.

7. Patient safety indicators will meet or exceed benchmark.

Boards often use benchmarks to track the organization's performance. Benchmarking can be applied in various ways. One way is to measure the organization's performance over time, comparing current activities to previous periods of time. Benchmarking may also include comparing the hospital's performance to nationally, regionally, or state-recognized performance goals or established industry targets. Many organizations use a combination of both types of benchmarking to understand how they are performing relative to best-in-class levels, as well as how the organization's performance has changed over time. The governing body fulfills its fiduciary responsibility by regularly meeting to review and analyze reports of the organization's progress toward its goals and benchmarks.

The board also oversees the hiring, supervision, and evaluation of the chief executive officer (CEO), who holds the highest employed role within the organization. Chief medical officers (CMOs) are often a close second in authority to the CEO. CEOs may have had many types of experiences in their professional preparation; some were physicians, some were chief operating officers (COOs). Originally some were chief financial officers (CFOs), others were chief nursing officers (CNOs), and some progressed from other positions in the health care industry. Many organizations also have a COO who is a part of the "C-Suite." The COO may oversee an entire organization or key components of the organization such as all clinical resources or nonclinical resources used within the organization. It is not uncommon for a CNO to report to a COO.

All CEOs have one thing in common: they are the visionary head of the organization, and they are responsible to the board for the overall performance of the organization. CEOs work with the board to set the organizational agenda and then track performance at the highest level through key performance indicators. These indicators usually fall into at least five categories including: clinical outcomes, finance, patient satisfaction, employee retention and performance, and growth.

Working with the CEO is a team of leaders who often have the descriptor "chief" or "vice president" as part of their title. Most organizations have a COO, who is responsible for all of the non-clinical resources used within the hospital, as well as the overall operations of the organization. The CFO is responsible for the budget, which includes the pricing of services, the collection of revenue, and the monitoring of budget to ensure capital purchases and fiscal stability. Organizations may also have attorneys as chief counsel, as well as vice presidents of marketing or planning or both; vice presidents of service or product lines, such as ambulatory services and cardiac care; vice presidents of facilities, human resources, fundraising (foundation), and so on.

Two other key roles are the CMOs and the CNO. The CMO is a physician who is ultimately responsible for all physician-related matters within the organization. CMOs often have business, health administration, or public health degrees in addition to a medical degree. The CMO is responsible for assisting the organized medical staff with physician appointments and credentialing, graduate medical education and continuing education, quality, and physician satisfaction. The CMO often works with a team of chiefs, who bear administrative responsibility for each of the clinical specialties, and medical directors, who are responsible for the clinical and administrative processes and quality within each specialty.

Hospital medical staffs are often comprised of a mix of physicians, physician assistants, nurse practitioners, and other individuals with high-level credentials. The medical staff may encompass private physicians, dentists, allied health professionals, full-time attending physicians, physicians with courtesy privileges, and faculty members. Over the past 10 years or more, services that are staffed 24/7 by physicians in positions such as intensivist, emergency medicine specialist, and hospitalist have emerged. As a result, hospitals have had to develop new rules and regulations pertaining to these roles. Although the primary function of medical staff bylaws is to describe the rules, regulations, responsibilities, and credentialing policies that apply to physicians and mid-level providers, this document is useful for nurse leaders as well, providing insight for nurses as they carry out the directions of the medical staff. The bylaws describe important elements of the chain of command, which may help nursing staff to communicate better and to feel secure in decisions they make as patient advocates. All medical staff leaders, including the CMO, play vital roles in the ongoing development and direction of the medical staff. Their interaction with nurse leaders helps to ensure the quality and safety of patient care.

Paralleling the medical staff's relationship with the CMO, the staff nurses have a leader who is ultimately responsible for the direction of the nursing organization. The CNO is a registered nurse who often has a master of science in nursing (MSN) degree as well as advanced training in business or health administration. Many CNOs and other nurse leaders also receive certification in nursing leadership through the American Nurses' Credentialing Center. CNOs have responsibility for all nursing-related patient care, and they often have additional areas of responsibility such as social work, pharmacy, laboratory, respiratory therapy, chaplaincy, and other services that work in tandem with nursing.

A hospital's nursing division accounts for the largest single discipline within the organization. In contrast to private physicians, who make rounds to check on their patients, and members of other services, who see patients at regular times during the course of their hospitalization, nursing is accountable for patient care 24/7. This incredibly valuable resource requires the utmost management due to its size and the complexity of its competencies. The biggest mistake nonclinicians make is to suppose "a nurse is a nurse is a nurse." We would never say the same thing about physicians. We know there is a vast difference between a cardiovascular surgeon and a psychiatrist. Recognizing and advocating for the various types of nursing roles, and the expertise and skills needed for each, is a crucial aspect of nursing leadership.

WHAT ARE THE OTHER TYPES OF NURSE LEADERS?

Working with the CNO are other vital staff members including directors of nursing, who oversee clinical and administrative areas such as emergency care, surgery, nursing education, nursing informatics, quality, and nursing research. Each director of nursing works with nurse managers, who are responsible for the daily operation of individual units. Within each unit, there may be charge nurses, shift leaders, team leaders, council leaders, and so on. Depending on the governance of the nursing organization (a topic we will discuss at length in chapter 4), there may also be leaders for clinical quality, professional ethics, research, resource allocation, and other types of councils. Beyond the leadership roles in group settings, there are also one-on-one leaders, such as peer mentors, nurse preceptors, and clinical resource specialists.

HOW ARE NURSE LEADERS PREPARING FOR THE FUTURE?

Opportunities for leadership in nursing abound. As a nurse leader, it is imperative to participate in establishing direction for the organization. It is also imperative that a nurse leader know the organization's strategic plan, the governing body's targets for performance, and the role that nursing is to play in achieving such goals.

At a higher level, nurse leaders also need to understand the future direction of the nursing industry in the United States. The role of nurses and the demographics of the nursing workforce are changing. In 2008, the federal government instituted new Medicare payment rules that would penalize organizations demonstrating poor performance on eight nursing-sensitive indicators. For the first time, hospital payment is tied to the quality of nursing care. This represents a sea of change for nurses, both in terms of the care they provide and the ways in which that care is documented. As a recent article in the *American Journal of Nursing* noted, managing nursing quality to achieve benchmark-level performance is not always easy.

> Among the challenges nurse leaders face is the relative lack of data on the quality of nursing care and inconsistencies among the evaluation tools used to measure care quality. These inconsistencies exist even among data collection initiatives focused on nursing performance, such as the National Database of Nursing Quality

Indicators (NDNQI) and the California Nursing Outcomes Coalition Database (CalNOC) Project. And they persist despite endorsement by the [National Quality Forum] NQF of Voluntary Consensus Standard for Nursing Sensitive Care.[3]

At the same time that the focus on quality is heating up, the face of nursing is changing significantly. A review of nurse staffing trends for the period 2000–2007 indicates that, while the current nursing shortage seems to have peaked in 2001, the short- and long-term implications of this shortage are still very much with us. In the short term, we are seeing a greater preponderance of older nurses—in part because of the large cohort of baby boomers who entered the nursing workforce in the 1970s and 1980s, and in part because the faltering economy has kept those persons in the workforce longer than anticipated. In 2007, registered nurses over the age of 50 were the fastest growing age group among the RN workforce, increasing 11% between 2003 and 2007.[4] The same study also found a growing trend toward foreign-born nurses, who represented over 30% of the total growth in RN employment during the same period.[4]

Over the long term, there are significant concerns about nursing education programs. In brief, program capacity is too small and the faculty too few to accommodate the growing need for nurses that the baby boom has created. Both the American Association of Colleges of Nursing and the National League for Nursing have noted that thousands of qualified applicants have been turned away from nursing programs because of space and faculty constraints.

The American Organization of Nursing Executives (AONE) recognizes that these issues create significant management challenges for nurse leaders. In the July 2004 issue of *Hospital and Health Networks* magazine, AONE's CEO, Pamela Thompson, noted:

> Even though we don't know what future patient care models will require, we have to act now. There is an old but familiar adage, "May you live in interesting times." Certainly, that applies to health care. Each day we are sculpting the shape of our future patient care delivery system, but its shape is ill-defined and we really don't know what it will look like in the end.[5]

We can make some assumptions. By 2010, there will be inadequate numbers of health care workers to deliver care using the same models that we use today. Advances in information management, therapeutics, and technology are dramatically altering the care required. Linear thinking is giving way as we embrace the science of chaos theory and complex adaptive systems.

These changes mean we have many questions about what the future will require, but we cannot wait until we have all the answers. We must begin to experiment and act now. One of the most important tasks is to define the work of the future; then we can identify the roles and competencies that we will need to do that work.

AONE continues to address these challenges. It created a task force to address the question: "What are the principles that can guide us as we define future patient care delivery models and who is the nurse who will be providing care to our patients in the future?" Out of this effort came seven principles that are now being disseminated in the hope they will stimulate conversations that will help define our future.

1. The actual work of nurses will change in the future, but the core values of caring and knowledge will remain.

2. The care provided will be decided in partnership with the patient.

3. The knowledge base of the nurse will shift from "knowing" a specific body of knowledge to "knowing how to access" the ever-changing information needed to manage care.

4. Processing the information accessed will expand the nurse's use of "critical thinking" to "critical synthesis," coordinating and negotiating care across multiple levels, disciplines, and settings.

5. The knowledge that is leveraged and the care provided are grounded in the relationships between the patient and the multidisciplinary team.

6. Relationships with patients will be dramatically altered by the increased application of technology, requiring that we further define the relationship context as being "virtual" or "physical" and know when each is required.

7. The ultimate future work of the nurse will be to partner with the patient or client to help him or her manage the individual journey of care.[5]

Although these seven principles may seem simple, they will become the platform for the conversations that will guide us as we sculpt the future.

> *"The ability to deal with ambiguity while developing physician relationships and partnerships [is] integral to the work of the nurse leaders. It is also important that leaders demonstrate work-life balance so that our young talented nurses will desire to move into leadership positions."*
>
> —Patricia Crome, RN, MN, CNA, FACMPE
> Principal, Rona Consulting Group; past member,
> AONE Board of Directors, Seattle, Washington.

CASE STUDY

Mercy Hospital is a community hospital with 250 inpatient beds. The facility provides care to a geographic distribution of 275 square miles. Mercy Hospital is a member of a system of 25 hospitals called Mercy Healthcare System (MHS). The MHS home office is centrally located in the upper Midwest; however, the 25 hospitals are located in four surrounding states.

After an intense strategic planning session, which included management from the system facilities as well as membership from the nearby community and local colleges, the governing body of MHS delivered the following strategic direction to its 25 hospitals and key leadership:

1. Bottom line: 3%+ net.
2. Installation of a centralized clinical documentation system within 36 months.
3. Ranking in the top 10% nationally for patient satisfaction using a nationally recognized tool.
4. Completion of a community benefits *pro forma* for community dissemination at the end of the fiscal year.
5. Employee satisfaction rating of 88% or higher.
6. Quality rating in the top 10% for the clinical indicators identified by the Center for Medicaid and Medicare Services (CMS).
7. Implementation of at least one strategy that results in new revenue.

Assessment Questions

1. Who are the key leaders in your organization, and how do they interact with each other and with the nursing staff?
2. What is your organization's mission and vision statement, and how do those statements influence leader decision making?
3. What are your organization's goals, and how do nurses help to achieve those goals?
4. What goals affect you directly?
5. What role will you play in assuring achievement of these goals?
6. What department-specific goals have you developed, and how have staff members assisted in development as well as achievement of these goals?
7. Describe the role you play in relationship to the medical staff and goal achievement.
8. Who are the nurse leaders in your organization, and how did they become leaders?
9. What are the opportunities to become a leader within your own organization?
10. How is leadership development encouraged and supported?

Best Practice

- Know who your leaders are, what they do as leaders, and how their leadership influences the organization.
- Know your organization's mission and vision, and how they influence leadership processes.
- Be knowledgeable about the organization's strategic directives and goals.
- Nursing leadership success requires regular interaction with the medical staff for communication, relationship building, goal achievement, goal development, and policy and practice changes.
- Always allow for ongoing feedback on ways to improve processes in your area as well as the organization as a whole. Use this feedback as a way to close the loop with staff and let them know you follow through.
- Recognize that leadership takes on many different forms and roles, both informal and formal.
- Remember that success as a leader takes time, support, and teamwork.
- Recognize the opportunities for leadership growth for yourself and others.
- Remember that leadership styles and functions may take many forms, but that all leadership should be aligned around common goals.

REFERENCES

1. Goleman, D. (1998). *Working with emotional intelligence.* New York, NY: Bantam Books.
2. American Hospital Association Resource Center. Fast Facts on U.S. Hospitals, 2009. Available at: http://www.aha.org/aha/resource-center/Statistics-and-Studies/fast-facts.html
3. Kurzman, E. T., & Buerhaus, P. I. (2008). New Medicare payment rules: Danger or opportunity for nursing? *American Journal of Nursing,108,* 30–35.

4. Buerhaus, P. I., Auerbach, D. I., & Staiger, D. O. (2007). Recent trends in the registered nurse labor market in the U.S: Short-run swings on top of long-term trends. *Nursing Economics, 25*, 59–66.
5. Thomson, P. (2004). Guiding principles. *Hospital and Health Networks, 78*(7), 86.

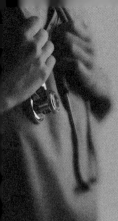

Chapter 2
FINANCE

"The overriding concern that keeps me up at night relates to the fiscal issues in health care. Of course, this is not a new issue and leaders have struggled with this dilemma for over 150 years. Every year local health care organizations provide over $20 million in care that is not reimbursed due to the uninsured—leaving only a 1% margin for staff development, salary increases, and capital investment. The Healthcare Association of New York reported in the spring of 2007, that 56 New York hospitals reported a 1% profit margin for the eighth straight year. In aggregate, 86% of New York hospitals had less than a 4% profit. At the same time, payers reported double-digit increases in premiums and reserves. Many of these payers reported several billion dollars in profits after meeting reserve requirements. Without a margin, there can be no mission. We must redesign health care insurance and Medicare."

—Deborah Zimmermann, RN, MS, NEA-BC,
Rochester, New York;
Board of Directors, Magnet Commission
Silver Spring, Maryland

WHAT IS FINANCE?

At its most basic, finance is the business side of health care. Finance covers a range of subject areas, including planning, budgeting, contracting, pricing, and purchasing. Many people who enter nursing say they do not like, or do not want to think about, the "numbers" side of what is traditionally a caring profession. Yet today more than ever, nurses and nurse leaders need to understand both what finance is, and the ways in which their roles as nurses have a bearing on financial outcomes.

Today's health care environment is the most complicated we have ever known. However, the current trend toward flattening organizational structures and using bottom-up planning means that we all need a certain degree of financial savvy in addition to our clinical nursing expertise.

TYPES OF BUDGETS

The most basic building block within finance is the budget. Most organizations have many types of budgets, from organization-wide operating budgets, to project-based budgets, to capital budgets for major developments. These budgets become the benchmarks for the various types of reporting that nurse leaders and their colleagues develop throughout the year.

Organizations may use various types of budgets, either alone or in tandem. These budgets include staffing, supply, operating, and capital budgets. The staffing budget is defined as the revenue and expense associate with the human resources necessary to provide the organization's services. Staffing may include clinical, nonclinical, professional, administrative, and support personnel.

The supply budget is defined as the revenue and expense associated with all of the consumable items needed to provide the organization's products and services. Both clinical and nonclinical items are included, so that items in the supply budget may include everything from oxygen, to photocopy paper, to blood products. Appropriate charge capture is exceedingly important to ensuring that the supply budget is both accurately projected and maintained.

The capital budget is defined as the revenue and expense associated with purchase of land, buildings, and equipment for operations that will not be resold and that have a useful life of more than 1 year, have a cost greater or equal to $500, and are subject to depreciation.[1]

The operating budget is defined as the revenue and expense associated with producing the organization's products and services.[2] Both the staffing budget and the supply budget roll up into the overall operating budget. Operating budgets typically include department- or service-line-specific budgets as well as an organization-wide operating budget.

HOW NURSE LEADERS USE BUDGETS

On a regular basis, often monthly, nurse leaders and the leadership team evaluate how funds come in and are spent in order to meet the organization's goals. The information compiled for an organizational budget and the associated ongoing reporting come from various sources. The most truly effective and engaging process is a "bottom-up" one, in which budget development, evaluation, and revision happen with the input of those working within the budgeted area, the end users. Within each unit, leaders and staff members use assessment tools to review and recommend budget items. The leadership then compiles the assessment reports as the basis for developing the annual budget.

HOW BUDGETING IS DONE

The budget cycle is usually the same every year, beginning 4 to 5 months before the beginning of the next fiscal year. This length of time allows for the necessary validation processes and governing board approval prior to implementation. In addition to the annual budget, many organizations develop a 3- to 5-year budget *pro forma* that can be used as a tool for the annual budgeting process as well as organizational strategic planning.

In developing a budget, the intent is to provide the best possible projections as to where the organization will be from one fiscal year to the next. The CEO/CFO, other key administrative staff, and key members of the governing body utilize both the annual and long-range budgets within the context of ongoing environmental assessments.

THE IMPORTANCE OF EXTERNAL FACTORS ON BUDGET DEVELOPMENT

For any budget, it is always important to begin with an environmental scan and share that with key leadership. For instance, in an annual budget, the environmental scan always focuses on the impact commercial payers will have on revenues. Do they plan to increase, stay neutral, or decrease payments? Similar questions ought to be determined for the Medicare population and their payments as well as the Medicaid program. Will your organization see more self-pay, uninsured, or underinsured patients? Will there be a change in the market (such as an increase in population or a shift in businesses that may have an impact on volumes)? Each of these elements must be factored into the environmental scan.

HOW THE CHANGING HEALTH CARE ENVIRONMENT AFFECTS TODAY'S BUDGETING

Given the current state of the U.S. economy, market and environment questions are vital to successful planning and budgeting. Notably, payers and the Centers for Medicare and Medicaid Services (CMS) are increasing their scrutiny of hospital pricing. No longer will they respond to the hospital's requirement to "pay more because it costs more than last year to provide the service." Furthermore, in the past, patients had little sensitivity about the cost of their care. As more employers lower the level of coverage they provide and institute high-deductible options, patients bear an increasing percentage of the payment burden.

Although questions relating to market and environment are closely linked with legal and policy sources, there can be no denying the impact they have on nursing. For instance, we have already seen a reduction in preventive and elective services as a result of the economy. Simply put, patients are going without services (including regular screenings, annual examinations, and medications) because of cost. When patients change their utilization patterns, as they have already done, hospitals see a shift in volume away from profitable services and an increase in emergency care. In the current economy, health care organizations have experienced a marked increase in uncompensated care of the indigent, and co-pays have become more and more difficult to collect. All of these trends, combined, have resulted in skyrocketing rates of bad debt and charity care.

Responding to the shift in utilization and the resulting financial impact is more than the job of the finance department. An effective response relies on the input of staff nurses and nursing leadership together with the entire health care team. In their role at the point of care, nurses interact with physicians, the hospital staff, and patients, all of whom have particular needs and agendas within the care process. Because of their intuitive capabilities, nurses are often the team members most able to identify needed resources to achieve the desired outcomes for all of those involved.

EVALUATING BUDGET REQUESTS

Given the very slim margins that exist today in health care, careful attention is necessary before purchasing expensive new equipment, developing new programs, or building projects. However, the staff, leadership, and physicians usually are aware of the latest advances in their practice—whether a new colleague will be joining their practice, whether care will be shifted from one setting to another, and so on—and so are often able to provide the context when recommending changes in the budget from one period to the next.

When considering large expenditures (e.g., over $500), many organizations require that a return on investment (ROI) study be done. Whether in the form of a simple worksheet or a full-blown business plan, an ROI tells leaders whether the investment will add value to the organization, and how quickly the investment will pay for itself. (An example of a budget worksheet is included with nursing leadership tools in the Appendix).

A similar exercise is necessary in order to place capital equipment on the budget. Budgeting should not be looked at as the development of a "wish list"; rather, it is truly a means to assess the needs of the organization for the next year as well as the few years beyond, thus assuring alignment with the organization's mission and strategic plan.

Although they may not seem to be connected, patient care models, physical plant, supply chain, and finance are all interwoven. When hospital leaders and architects design the environment of care, they must think through issues and questions relating to these factors together. For example: Is the patient care unit centralized so that the rooms surround the nursing station or are there long hallways that cause the staff much lost time going back and forth to the station? Is the nursing station decentralized; that is, are all of the resources such as medications, linen, scales, supplies, and other necessary items located in "pods" throughout the unit? If supplies and equipment are not easy to access, they will not be used efficiently. (Put another way, a large bandage that is within arm's reach is much more likely to be used than a smaller, more cost-efficient bandage stored 20 feet away). With the increasing acuity of patients, shorter lengths of stay, and greater use of less invasive care technology, staff is under constant pressure to work as efficiently as possible at the bedside. Inefficiencies may lead to hoarding of items, patient safety concerns, communication problems, and other factors that ultimately drive up costs within the unit and the organization.

Therefore, up-front modeling and assessments are important measures to ensure budgeting and cost-efficiency. Unit and department leaders use these assessments to understand how changes in processes and programs will change patient days of care, lengths of stay, and technology and equipment use, as well as staffing, supplies, and operations. For the nurse leader, this information is key to developing the staffing, supply, capital, and operations budgets.

Once these assessments are complete, the finance department assimilates these assessments into a single budget for the entire organization. This assimilation is performed with the assistance of materials management, information technology (IT), and human resources leadership. These assimilated documents constitute a "first pass" at what the net fiscal year will look like. This due diligence is the most important step of the budgeting process. Before being finalized, budgets are often revised and reworked to ensure that under- and overprojections do not occur.

WORKING WITH FINALIZED BUDGETS

Once the due diligence process is complete and approved by the governing board, each organizational leader receives his or her approved budget "packet." This final budget is then the benchmark that is used to assess how well the unit is managed based on the staffing and salary projections as well as the operational data, which includes the number of admissions, length of stay, and total days of care. Days of care can be converted into visits for such areas as ambulatory units (e.g., an emergency department or clinic) or treatments for an infusion center or dialysis unit.

Many organizations use a formal, unit-based reporting tool to track the ongoing success of each department. When used by both unit staff and leaders, this "report card" also provides an opportunity to assess for variances and the ability to analyze such variances. For example, how would a unit staff use their report card to evaluate the loss experienced when a key provider moves out of the area? Assuming that no replacement is found for the individual, they would be able to track the impact of his or her leaving by studying changes in their budget (which had not been anticipated when the budget was developed prior to the provider's move). If the key provider performed at least 16 surgeries per month with an average length of stay of 3 days, this move could lead to a decrease of 48 days of expected care, as well the loss of revenue associated with that care. Analyzing this kind of data allows leadership to develop an action plan to address variances and manage expenses accordingly.

FINANCE CHANGES OVER THE PAST 25 YEARS

Health care finance has changed dramatically over the past 25 years. Hence, the preceding description does not reflect the processes that nurse leaders performed in years past. Although basic budgeting is now recognized as a minimal competency, most nursing education provides little preparation for financial competencies. Thus, many nurse leaders find themselves learning finance as part of their staff positions.

The changes that we have experienced over time are myriad. Twenty-five years ago, the nurse leader would provide a handwritten document to the materials management department noting that only a few capital items were necessary. Such items might include a wheelchair or several intravenous poles. The unit nursing leadership would also provide human resources with a handwritten document noting projected staffing needs, called a "master budget," for the next fiscal year. These needs were based on known departures from employment or extended leaves of absence. Because both the clinical models of care and the hospital revenue models were simpler, patients had longer lengths of stay and occupancy was much higher. Thus, factors like admissions, lengths of stay, and patient turnover were not given consideration in the budgeting process.

With a predefined operating margin (usually 2% to 5%), the fiscal, materials management, and human resource departments would compile the data and provide it to the CEO. The CEO would then, in collaboration with the CFO, scrub it if necessary and provide the revised data to the governing board for approval and implementation for the beginning of the next fiscal year. Nursing involvement was minimal because the role of nursing in leadership and the administrative processes of the hospital were separated into a much greater degree than they are now.

However, over time, revenue models became more complex. With the advent of managed care and sophisticated government and private health care payment systems, hospitals experienced pressure to lower lengths of stay and reduce costs per case. Operating margins have shrunk over the past two decades, so that many organizations are running with little or no excess. Budgeting is vital to ensure the right amount of personnel, equipment, and supplies for variation in patient demand.

NURSING INVOLVEMENT IN BUDGET MANAGEMENT

Similarly, recent emphasis on patient safety and quality, as well as the Centers for Medicaid and Medicare Services' scrutiny of adverse events means that every element of the patient care process must now be planned for, closely monitored, and scrutinized for efficiency.

Today, the sophistication of these processes requires nurse leaders to have a significant amount of competence in order to facilitate the multi-million dollar budgets they direct. It is also imperative that the frontline staff understand their role in budget adherence. For example, it is very easy for a fiscal staff member to assess the budget in relationship to the current environment and determine that in order to achieve the budget goals, at least $1 million in expenses needs to be reduced from the budget. If a nurse leader were to say the same thing to a staff nurse, the staff nurse would initially indicate she or he would assist in this endeavor. Missing from that scenario, however, is the specific direction and means for the individual nurse to achieve this goal. If, on the other hand, the staff nurse was told to ensure careful monitoring of 10 items with the highest unit cost, or to ensure quick reporting of broken or lost equipment, that nurse would have specific and incremental ways of working to keep the budget on track.

Nurse leaders need (and should use) objective tools to provide the necessary direction to the frontline staff. For instance, suppose a medical/surgical unit was asked to reduce expenses by $1 million. What would that look like? What types of less expensive supplies could be eliminated or substituted? What impact would reducing the length of stay by 1 day or even 6 hours have on the overall expenses and resources? What effect might reassessing the drug profile have? Or is there vast variation in treatment protocols among the care providers? Many opportunities exist at the point of care to examine such questions, and the staff nurses can assist in playing a major role in achieving the resulting objectives.

The American Nurses Credentialing Center's Magnet Recognition Program®, which demonstrates best practice as well as identifying high-performing organizations, emphasizes that nursing organizations must be continually assessed, and appropriate strategic and quality plans for nursing and patient care developed. The CNO is responsible for securing adequate resources to implement these plans through the engagement of interdisciplinary efforts. Today, more than ever before, the fiscal department is an integral partner with the nursing division.

REVENUE

Expense is only one side of the health care business equation. There is also the revenue side, which includes money received for providing patient care and other sorts of income (such as money from the sale of bonds, loans, donations, and grants, all of which comprise so-called nonpatient service revenue). Revenue may be prospective, meaning that a prenegotiated amount of money is paid in anticipation of the amount of service provided, or it may be reimbursed, meaning it is paid after the service is rendered and a filed claim has been approved for payment. Organizations negotiate rates of payment for the services they provide with third-party payers. Some of these rates are set by federal and state sources. Others, like those for local commercial payers, are negotiated on a regular basis. The work of determining payment is a combination of history, science, and art.

Most pricing and payment models trace their origin to the Medicare system, the insurance plan established by the federal government in 1965 to pay for health care for U.S. citizens 65 years of age and older.* Subsequently, the CMS (formerly called the Health Care Financing Authority) recognized that rather than simply paying hospitals what they billed, a standardized method of documenting and paying for the care provided to Medicare patients was needed. In the early 1970s the U.S. government commissioned a think tank at Yale University to develop such a system. The result was the development of the diagnostic related groups (DRGs) model, which organizes care into major diagnostic categories such as cardiac or surgical care. Based on actuarial data, these groups were assigned a weight determining the payment and an average length of stay for each type of care. The Medicare DRGs predefined reimbursement, and since their development, all adjustments to payment rates have worked off the original DRG base rate. Because the DRGs acted and continue to function as the foundation for payment, health care organizations had to put together mechanisms to monitor and manage patients whose care was paid for in this way.

DRGs continue to be the coding means used to document and bill for care, whether provided through Medicare or other insurance providers. Other payers in the marketplace include the commercial insurance groups such as Aetna, Blue Cross, and Blue Shield; state-administered Medicaid programs; and military insurance such as TriCare. Although administered

---

*Because of increases in the number of Medicare participants and concerns about the future ability to sustain this federally funded health care program, significant efforts are currently underway to address this situation. Many questions can be answered at their Web site www.medicare.gov.

through separate programs, these sources of revenue have an impact on each other.

Over time, the adjustments to Medicare rates have not kept up with the cost of providing care. Changes in technology, models of care, and staffing have driven up costs faster than the federal government could keep pace. At the same time, the U.S. population has aged so that more patients now have Medicare as their primary insurance. Additionally, older patients tend to use more health care services than younger patients. These three factors add up to more patients using more care, but at a lower rate of reimbursement than it costs to provide that care.

Health care organizations have responded to this deficit by "cost shifting," a process whereby pricing is increased overall so that payers other than Medicare absorb the difference in reimbursement to cover the gap. Commercial payers understand this activity, which is implied in payment discussions that use terms such as "120% of Medicare." However, the general public may not understand this concept. Hospital administrators are not being greedy; they are simply trying to balance out the revenue sources to ensure that they can provide care to the total patient population in a cost-efficient way. Thus, ongoing data within the finance department provides the information necessary for the negotiation process involving rate adjustments from commercial payers other than Medicare.

This type of balancing cannot continue forever, and over the years, providers and payers have tried many different models to ensure that high-quality care is given at a reasonable rate. Most health care leaders recognize that there are two dynamics at play: On the one hand, there is the need for local quality management and cost control. That need has led to the creation of health maintenance organizations (HMOs), disease management programs, and various types of employer-driven risk-sharing programs. However, we also recognize a need for reform on the national level. At issue is the fact that the base methodology for DRGs, established nearly 40 years ago, is not the best model for how care is given today.

When the diagnostic groups were weighted back in the 1970s, they were calculated using both clinical data about how care is rendered and geographic data about the cost of providing care in different regions of the United States. Using these cost-based DRGs, a total hip replacement performed in Tampa, Florida, would be paid at a different rate than one in New York City, or Bismarck, North Dakota. At the time, the variations in cost made sense; however, as incremental increases have been made, they have historically been instituted as a percentage of the base rate. Thus, if the same care is reimbursed at $100, $150, or $50 (depending on location), a 3% increase in payment shifts the rates to $103, $154.50, and $51.50. Over time, these incremental increases are compounded. The result is that significant disparities in payment now exist. On the other hand, disparities in cost are not that significant. For example, if a hospital were to purchase a 64-slice computed tomography scanner, the cost for the equipment and supplies would be pretty much the same no matter where in the United States the facility was located. Thus, the inequity of payment versus cost has become a problem for health care, in general.

In North Dakota, where I work, the reimbursement model was identified as a significant problem. Over an 8-year period, stakeholders from around the state worked to develop stronger relationships with their congressional delegation and to educate them about the impact of this model on the provision of health care in the state. Employees, community members, and local, regional, and state leadership all came together for this effort in an attempt to align payment for care in North Dakota with that of regional peer organizations and rural states. Ultimately the state's hospitals received a 3-year reprieve relating to the reimbursement provided, and subsequently, the reimbursement model was reweighted. The reweighting, however, has not kept pace with the associated inflation.

Communication and relationship development are key components of the payer negotiation processes. Nurse leaders help by communicating budgeting needs and participating in internal review processes to ensure cost efficiency. They help externally by working with contracting staff, administration, and external parties (including payers, hospital trade associations, and professional organizations) to evaluate and revise payment policies.

In addition to patient service revenue, other sources of revenue are determined by the Medicare cost report that each health care organization is required to submit annually to the federal government. This report provides a financial "picture" of the organization. It also determines whether the organization is eligible for additional funding to augment patient service revenue.

There are three additional funding sources: (1) disproportionate share hospital (DSH) funds, (2) graduate medical education (GME) funds, and (3) so-called "refund" payments. DSH funds are funds that are paid to hospitals with a payer mix that has a consistently high percentage of persons on Medicare and Medicaid; GME funds are funds that are paid to hospitals to offset the costs incurred in training medical residents; and a "refund" payment is a payment from Medicare for overpayment by the medical facility during a defined fiscal year. Because each of these revenue types is based on special circumstances surrounding the patient care provided by the individual hospital, each hospital has to substantiate its ongoing eligibility for the funding through volume, payer mix, case mix, and teaching programs.

Bad debt and charity care are also fundamental facts of business for health care organizations. Not-for-profit organizations are required by the federal government to demonstrate their value to the community from care that is rendered without payment and other intangible services. The care that is provided without payment falls into two categories: write-offs of uncollectible charges and uncompensated care of the indigent (known collectively as bad debt and charity care). The intangible services may not be clinical care per se, but fall under the umbrella of community programs such as health fairs and blood pressure clinics.

Further, not-for-profit organizations must show how they use any "profit" (i.e., revenue in excess of expense) to invest in organizational improvements, such as technology, equipment, construction, or renovation. Depending on the location and type of organization, the amount of bad debt and charity care may vary significantly. However, all organizations are required to publicly disclose their bad debt and charity care through annual reports. Inner-city organizations often have a higher rate of bad debt and charity care, as well as DSH payments.

As yet another example of how health care finance has changed in the past decade, approaches to bad debt and charity care are also evolving. However, as coverage models shift to create higher deductibles and co-pays, all organizations bear the responsibility of maximizing payment capture and collection systems so that revenue due to the organization is not lost unnecessarily. Whereas these topics were hardly mentioned in administrative discussions 10 years ago, nurse leaders now participate in many projects to improve charge capture and secure up-front payment for services.

UNDERSTANDING THE TENSION BETWEEN FINANCE AND PATIENT CARE

Although many nurse leaders have welcomed the opportunity to participate in discussions about health care budgets, revenue, and cost containment, not all of these conversations have gone smoothly. Whenever an organization examines how to protect its operating margins, questions about the quality of care and approaches to caring are sure to follow. Some may even go so far as to raise the question of which is most important, advocating for the needs of the patient or respecting the needs of the organization. The myriad of changes that have occurred over the past decade, including federal reductions and freezes in funding, changes in coding requirements, and increased financial risk associated with adverse events, have continued to highlight the relationship and tension between patient care and finance.

In fact, the dynamic is not a question of "either/or" (either patient care or profitability), rather, it is a matter of appropriate payment for appropriate care. When viewed in that light, the challenge facing health care providers spotlights the pivotal role of nurse leaders in creating and maintaining modern approaches to patient care. Nurse leaders have helped to create a picture of a three-legged stool, with reimbursement as one leg, quality and patient safety as another, and public reporting and transparency as the third. None of these legs exists in isolation; in fact, they are very interdependent. The federal governments as well as private insurers are demanding improved performance and greater consistency in how organizations provide care by asking health care providers to demonstrate excellence in these areas. Nurse leaders can help to draw out the interdependencies among these three areas and clarify the way in which appropriate payment can be made for appropriate care.

Not only are organizations expected to do more with less, they are also expected to provide care at a lower cost and higher quality than payers had demanded years ago. In this context, nurse leaders help to identify, implement, and document outcomes measures and evidence-based practice, so that insurers will contract with the organization at favorable rates. Without that level of monitoring and service reporting, organizations may miss opportunities to improve payment, and insurers may require their beneficiaries to seek care elsewhere.

EXTERNAL REPORTING AND PUBLIC ACCOUNTABILITY

The majority of U.S. hospitals are not-for-profit, meaning that the organizations do not pay taxes and any operating surplus is expected to be reinvested in the organization. Not-for-profit systems are required by law to provide free care to the indigent. Many public hospitals (those that are owned by the county or state in which they operate) also function as primary residency programs for medical schools.

Today, not-for-profit organizations are under increasing scrutiny to account for the care they provide. Given the increases in health care cost and growing awareness of quality, the public is demanding that not-for-profit hospitals demonstrate their value to the community. Every year, hospitals must publish audited financial statements for the previous fiscal year, as well as file a Form 990 with the Internal Revenue Service, which reports on the organization's financial activities. All not-for-profit hospital 990s are available to the public via the Web site http://www.guidestar.gov. Tools such as Catholic Health Association's Charity Care reporting tool help member organizations and others comply with the necessary reporting of the community benefit they provide through free care, screening activities, educational programs, and other efforts to improve the health and welfare of those most at risk.

Recent federal legislation, such as the Sarbanes-Oxley Act of 2002, increased the accountability and transparency of both not-for-profit and investor-owned organizations. The same rigor is necessary today. Hospitals cost communities in two ways—through the payments they receive in Medicaid (which is partially state funded), and because they do not pay taxes on their land or assets. Therefore, the community has a right to know that its investment is being used wisely.

FEDERAL AUDITING AND PAY-FOR-PERFORMANCE IMPACT

The federal government is the largest health care payer, through its Medicaid and Medicare programs. With the aging and retirement of the baby boomers, health care faces a growing crisis; this cohort will significantly increase the number of people who will become Medicare-eligible while, at the same time, fewer workers will be paying into the Medicare trust fund. Furthermore, when the Medicare program was created, the average life expectancy was much shorter than it is today. Consequently, the average Medicare beneficiary is using services over a longer period of time than the program's developers originally anticipated.

Medicare payment rules are very complex, and it is quite easy for organizations to misapply those rules in their coding and billing of patient care. In 2003, Congress directed the

Department of Health and Human Services (DHHS) to conduct a 3-year demonstration program using recovery audit contractors (RACs) to detect and correct improper payments in the Medicare fee-for-service program. The RAC demonstration program was designed to determine whether the use of these audits would be a cost-effective means of protecting the Medicare trust fund by minimizing inappropriate payments to providers and suppliers.

The RACs are paid a percentage of the audited savings they identify through their audits. Depending on what the auditors find, hospitals may have to reimburse CMS for funds that were paid inappropriately. Nursing has a key role to play in these audits, in helping to ensure the appropriate resource utilization and charge capture so coding inconsistencies and billing problems are minimized.

As mentioned in chapter 1, the U.S. government is also increasing its scrutiny of care to prevent payment for conditions that were caused or exacerbated by hospital care. Such items include catheter-associated urinary tract infections, pressure ulcers, hospital-acquired infections, deemed "never events," as well as sentinel events that occur due to error. Patients entering the hospital do not expect to leave with additional injuries, infections, or other serious conditions that occur during the course of stay. Although some of these complications may be unavoidable, too often, patients suffer from injuries or illnesses that could have been prevented if the hospital had taken proper precautions.

On February 8, 2006, President Bush signed the Deficit Reduction Act (DRA) of 2005. Section 5001(c) of the DRA requires the Secretary to identify conditions that are (1) high cost or high volume or both, (2) result in the assignment of a case to a DRG that has a higher payment when present as a secondary diagnosis, and (3) could reasonably have been prevented through the application of evidence-based guidelines. Section 5001(c) provides that CMS can revise the list of conditions from time to time.

As part of its commitment to improve the quality of care patients receive during a hospital stay, and to make sure that Medicare only pays for items and services that are reasonable and necessary, Medicare is taking new steps to make hospitals safer by adopting payment policies that will encourage hospitals to (1) reduce the likelihood of hospital-acquired conditions and (2) reduce preventable medical errors, such as wrong-sided surgery.

Nurses play a major role in the prevention of problems that could lead to Medicare scrutiny. The initial intake assessment of the patient is vitally important to determine whether certain conditions are present when the patient arrives at the organization. The nurse at the point of care must document all assessment findings so that in the event, conditions such as an ulcer is present on admission, the organization does not get financially penalized for the treatment and expense associated with the condition during the hospitalization.

> *"The financial competency is often the one that is the scariest for new nursing leadership. The development of learning tools as well as ongoing mentoring and support provides the greatest opportunity for growth and development in this area. As a CNO, I recognize that I need to stay very close to new leaders and assist them at a minimum through two budget cycle processes."*
>
> — Terry Watne, MS, RN; Administrative Director, Altru Health System, Grand Forks, North Dakota

CASE STUDY

Donna Jacobs, RN, is the charge nurse for a 16-bed surgical unit. The 51-bed surgical unit has two nursing stations. One is located at the east end of the fourth floor and the other is at the west end of the same floor. Donna's responsibility is to monitor and manage patient flow, resources, quality, and safety. Within that overall job responsibility is managing staff overtime, general staff expenses, supply utilization and expenses, and patient length of stay. The most common diagnosis on this unit is the total joint patient. Based on historical trends, the length of stay for patients undergoing total knee replacement is about 2.5 days, and for patients undergoing total hip replacement averages 2.8 days. Within this context, the total number of patient care beds is 51 with an average daily census of 37 patients and a daily admission/discharge/transfer (ADT) rate of 75%. Regardless of acuity, each RN is responsible for four patients, and each nurse's aide assists the RN with 8 patients.

 Assessment Questions

1. What further impact can the charge RN have on expense reduction?
2. What means could be used to achieve this reduction?
3. Has the unit performed an indepth assessment such as a time and motion study to assess exactly what is occurring at what point in time during a typical surgical day? What are the findings? Are there redundancies? Are there functions that can be fulfilled by a staff member other than a highly skilled professional? What role can technology play in further reducing expenses? What role can the patient or family play in the patient's care and recovery process? What role does the medical staff play in this process? And finally, what quality and fiscal indicators will provide staff with the information that affirms the work they are doing is the right work? Are there benchmark celebration times? How is something like this sustained?
4. What leadership role can the charge nurse play in developing the same level of financial awareness in all of the line staff so that everyone works toward, and achieves, a common goal?

Best Practice

- Provide staff with data and the information necessary to achieve goals.
- Develop a mechanism so that an ongoing assessment of the goals and level of achievement of the goals are recognized.
- Develop teams made up of stakeholders in the goal so that the process is collaborative.
- Include finance staff for their expertise.
- Low cost/high quality being the goal, think outside the box to achieve these goals. At one time, a mother stayed in the hospital for 4 days after a normal vaginal delivery; now the typical stay is 2 days. What can be learned from that process, and how can the health care team play a role before and after surgical procedures or medical admission to assist in the care trajectory.

REFERENCES

1. Nowicki, M. (2001). *The financial management of hospitals and healthcare organizations* (p. 23). Chicago, IL: Healthcare Administration Press.
2. Nowicki, M. (2001). Glossary. In *The financial management of hospitals and healthcare organizations*. Chicago, IL: Healthcare Administration Press.

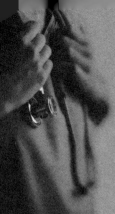

Chapter 3

QUALITY AND PATIENT SAFETY

"Leaders who are visible and regularly coach staff about the importance of quality and patient safety use this kind of role modeling to create and sustain environments that uphold expected behaviors and outcomes. The use of collaborative reward and recognition programs also contributes to 'team successes' and enhances best practices and quality patient outcomes."

—Cindy Lefton, RN, PhD;
Vice President Organizational Consulting,
Psychological Associates,
St. Louis, Missouri

WHAT IS QUALITY?

In the early 1930s, W. Edwards Deming and Joseph Juran worked at Western Electric Laboratories. They realized that complex production processes can often lead to variation. In order to improve quality, Deming and Juran recognized the need to decrease variation. Deming said, "Quality begins in the Boardroom." This is a simple way of saying that an orientation to quality begins at the top, if it is to be present throughout the organization. Deming and Juran developed a way of thinking about and working through production processes to improve consistency and raise quality. Their methods were most notably applied in manufacturing, and, in fact, they are often credited with rebuilding the Japanese manufacturing industry.[1]

Others have expanded on Deming and Juran's work by noting the other elements that influence variation. David Straker said that "quality means understanding. It means understanding people, what they value and, how they effectively trade with others. And it means working out how these imperfect systems can be optimized so our businesses thrive."[2]

HOW DO NURSES AFFECT HEALTH CARE QUALITY?

Everyone agrees that the goal of each health care provider is to deliver high-quality care. The question that we find harder to answer is, what does "quality" actually mean? For example, if someone were to ask whether quality care was provided or whether you, as a nurse, provided quality care, your first resounding response would be, "Of course, I provide quality care." However, the follow-up question, "How do you know you provide quality care?" might give you pause. In order to identify our perceptions of quality, we need to understand the tools and indicators we seek to measure.

One nurse might say, "I provide medications in a timely manner," with time being the measure. Another might say, "With my assessment skills, I am able to proactively assess my patients' conditions, notify the physician of variances, and provide the appropriate interventions." (In that case, she or he is measuring appropriateness as the indicator of quality.) Another nurse might say, "Feedback from patients, families, physicians, and colleagues indicates that the care I provide my patients and families is excellent." That nurse is using feedback and opinion scores to measure performance. There are numerous means to demonstrate quality in providing care. Measurement of quality can be qualitative or quantitative, or both. Numerous tools exist to measure quality and allow individuals, organizations, and the public to speak to the level of quality that exists. These tools also help users to develop plans for improving important aspects that may not meet a certain level of quality. Today more than ever, databases have been created to serve as clearinghouses or as a means to benchmark organizations with other organizations. Benchmarking assists in defining where opportunities exist as well as where a certain focus could occur. Some benchmark sets look at clinical indicators, while others look at structural and process indicators. Further, some benchmark data sets are nursing or service line specific, while others measure the entire team or organization.

Every nurse, from novice to expert, graduate nurse to chief nursing officer, has a direct responsibility for patient care quality. Nurse leaders have two roles: to provide the resources for high-quality care, and to continuously assess their own area of responsibility for quality improvement opportunities. Therefore, nurse leaders must be competent in both the theories behind quality improvement and the implementation of quality improvement tools and systems.

It is important to note that not all quality improvement projects must be overwhelming processes, nor do nurses (or their leaders) drive these processes alone. Because the quality of care is as complex as the care itself, improving the care you provide is best done with a multidisciplinary team determining which important aspects of care ought to be measured to ensure that quality care is being provided. Again, these aspects can be structured aspects, process aspects, and outcome aspects. Structure and process aspects influence outcomes. Therefore, knowing what outcome is desired and then measuring the structure or process, or both, can assist in ensuring that desired outcome(s) are achieved.

QUALITY PROCESS MONITORING

Process monitoring helps users determine whether the various steps in a process are occurring as anticipated to achieve the desired outcome. Medication administration is one of the most frequently cited areas for quality improvement and process monitoring, not only because of the growing number of medications in use, but also because of the many hand-offs that occur in the medication administration process. If the process of medication administration is not followed consistently, it might lead to medication errors, delays in treatment, and other problems for the patient. It also creates problems for the organization because such process glitches will likely lead to increased cost. Therefore, the nurse or nurse leader monitoring a medication administration process will want to ensure that the right drug is delivered intact, at the right time, and that the intended outcome of the drug e.g., pain relief occurs. Whether the medication is delivered intact is a structure measure, which will be discussed in the next section.

One of the most important elements of medication administration is timeliness. When the medication is administered is often as important as which medication and the dose that is used. If it is found that the medication is not being provided at the right time, evaluating the causes might lead to changes that will achieve timely administration. One possible cause might be conflicts in patient care scheduling. For instance, during the course of a patient's stay in the hospital, it is not uncommon for an ancillary team member to schedule a test or therapy during the same time medication ought to be administered. This time conflict could have an impact on the timeliness and effect of the medication administration, especially in regimens that include pain management, anticoagulant therapy, or insulin therapy. Process monitoring can be a very valuable means to determine whether the goals (and quality) of care are being achieved.

QUALITY STRUCTURE MONITORING

Structure monitoring is a means to assess the various items that allow a process to work. Structures may include computer programs, hospital equipment, or even room layout. One easy way to differentiate structures from processes is to recognize that once they are set up, structures stay relatively constant. For instance, once a lamp is put into a room, it will cast light—regardless of the wattage of bulb that is put into the lamp—when turned on. Without light as a structure in that room (a patient room, an operating room, or an office), the process intended for that room will not happen well (or at all). The key to structure monitoring is figuring out where to place the structure, how to use it, and where it fits in the process.

To explore this distinction further, we can go back to the example of medication administration. One very common structure in medication administration is storage. Many medications require careful storage in order to achieve their desired effects. Keeping a medication intact, meaning, in the state in which it is the most effective, becomes as important as figuring out the dosage and timing of administration. Regardless of how many patients receive that medication, it needs to be at a consistent temperature every time it is given. Therefore, monitoring the storage system to ensure that it is working properly and maintaining the desired temperature becomes an important structural measure. If the medication is refrigerated, for example, one might monitor whether the refrigerator stays within the target range of 34 to 40°F. A simple temperature log can provide the documentation necessary to ensure that such monitoring is in place.

Another way to think about structure monitoring is to recognize that the answer to a question about structure should not vary; it is usually a "yes/no" answer. "Is the refrigerator temperature at the desired temperature at 12 midnight every night?" In the event the answer is no, more in-depth analysis is needed. Perhaps in the course of monitoring the temperature, you notice that there are peak periods when the refrigerator is opened frequently, thereby raising the internal temperature. This would lead to two types of questions. The first would be a structural question: "Should we think about a different type of refrigerator that can withstand frequent opening and closing more easily?" The second would be a process question, and may be the simpler, quicker, and less expensive question to ask: "Can we change the process so that we don't need to open the refrigerator as often?" The preceding scenario is very similar to the process a surveyor from the Joint Commission on Accreditation of Healthcare Organizations might use during an accreditation visit.

At all times, with both process and structure monitoring, the care of the patient is the most important outcome to consider. Although many of the measures that go into quality improvement are predetermined by federal, state, and accrediting regulatory bodies, there are also numerous measures that can be chosen and studied by the patient care team. It is always a good idea to clarify what best practice indicates as a benchmark, and to ensure that the organization's leadership is aware of the process being studied and the benchmarks being used.

Benchmarking is a means to measure an indicator, a process, or an outcome against industry standards. These measures may have been set based on best practices, research, or both. Often, however, such "official" benchmarks do not exist; in these cases, a benchmark may be a self-established goal that one is attempting to achieve. Once the goal is achieved, the benchmark can be raised; therefore, "benchmarking against yourself" becomes the benchmark measurement. This process is similar to that used by an athlete who establishes a goal such as running a marathon in 3 hours or less. "Three hours or less" becomes the individual's goal and, when achieved, his or her "personal best." The next time that individual runs a marathon, he or she will attempt to exceed the current "personal best" and establish a new one.

Many tools and techniques are used to measure health care quality, and many of them have been written about, debated, and revised over time. Nurse leaders may find it useful to have a resource that can describe which tool is most helpful and effective in helping them think through the various types of quality studies that can be done—everything from root cause analysis to fishbone diagrams—as well as to enlist the help of leadership in working through large quality improvement projects. One easy way for any nurse to begin reducing variation and improving quality is by asking "why" five times. The following example shows how that exchange might play out in an operating room situation:

Q: Why do we find different recovery rates in our implant patients?

A: Because we are using three different types of implant devices, all with differing outcomes.

Q: Why do we use three types of implant devices?

A: Because Dr. Jones and Dr. O'Connor like type A, Dr. Smith likes type B, and Dr. Yates and Dr. Homs like type C.

Q: Why do they each like those types?

A: Those were the types they were trained to use in residency.

Q: Why don't we study the outcomes for each type of implant and compare them to what the literature indicates or recommends?

A: The evidence indicates that types A and C have the best outcomes and type B has moderate outcomes. We found that Dr. Smith prefers B but will use A on occasion.

Q: Why not speak to Dr. Yates about changing device preferences (based on the evidence) and then see if we can negotiate volume discounts with the group purchasing organization on the remaining two devices?

A: In these kinds of situations, the data obtained can be viewed as providing a picture of the individual's practice in relationship to that of other members of the team. This picture can be helpful when introducing the opportunity for change.

"We need to act with more speed and diligence to stop practice where it is actively harmful," Dr. Don Berwick said. "Let the need of the patient come first, not the need of the hospital."[3] As the preceding example shows, simply asking the question "why?" five times in a row can help an organization gain a clearer picture about why processes and structures are set up as they are, and how, over time, those very same elements have led to current results.

The American Nurses Association developed a definition of "nurse sensitive indicators" identifying them as "indictors that reflect the structure, process, and outcomes of nursing care."[4] Patient falls exemplify a situation in which nursing actions can have an impact on outcomes. A significant amount of research has been conducted relative to patient falls. Benchmarking for patient falls is also available. For nurses, studying the literature, studying the data for an organization surrounding patient falls, and establishing standards of practice offer a means to influence the effect of this nurse sensitive indicator on patient outcomes. Other nurse sensitive indicators can include pressure ulcers, infections, and use of restraints, all of which contribute to patient care outcomes.

QUALITY, PATIENT SAFETY, AND THE PUBLIC'S CALL FOR ACCOUNTABILITY

In addition to the efforts being made by those within the health care system to improve quality, the public increasingly is calling for transparency and quality improvement. In the past decade, reports from federal and national organizations such as the Institute of Medicine (IOM), the Institute for Healthcare Improvement, and the Commonwealth Fund have brought questions of health care quality and accountability into the open. Years ago, patients, the public, and payers simply expected each hospital and each provider to render the best care possible. Because of changing reimbursement, advances in health care practice, and the increasing complexity surrounding patient care, we now know that quality differs significantly based on where and when it is provided.

Patient advocates, payers, and others have raised a common theme in calling for increased provider accountability and transparency regarding the quality of patient care. Many organizations, including risk management insurers, payers, state credentialing bodies, the federal government, and not-for-profit advocacy groups, now require hospitals to report specific measures of quality. Great strides have been taken nationally to measure and develop transparency in reporting about the health care system's ability to provide quality patient care. This quality reporting system allows organizations as well as the public to evaluate organizations nationwide. Some of the organizations that evaluate and report on quality include Leap Frog, Health Grades, Thomson Reuters, and *U.S. News & World Report*. In the nursing industry, the National Database of Nursing Quality Indicators is a well-regarded reporting source used by Magnet-designated hospitals and other facilities that want to monitor nursing-sensitive quality measures.

Hospital governing boards are increasing their awareness as well; a recent study published in the *Journal of Healthcare Management* highlighted the direct correlation between having a board quality committee and the likelihood of adopting various oversight practices and achieving lower mortality rates for six common medical conditions measured by the Agency for Healthcare Research and Quality's Inpatient Quality Indicators and the State Inpatient Databases.[5]

Based on the systems that governing boards are putting into place, hospitals and their leaders now have a more comprehensive, consistent forum in which to examine their performance. When scores are out of range, the hospital leadership can systematically evaluate the data and report a plan as to how performance will improve, to the board. Governing boards are requiring that sophisticated reporting systems be put in place and that ongoing monitoring and evaluation occur so that in the event a score is out of range, the process of drilling down, investigating, and making changes, if necessary, can be completed in a relatively short, i.e., acceptable period of time.

QUALITY ACROSS ORGANIZATIONAL DOMAINS

It is important that organizations acknowledge the various systems, processes, and outcomes that most influence patient quality and focus their resources on achieving optimal performance. Nurse leaders are well advised to bear in mind both the high-volume and low-volume patient care types, and how their respective clinical and resource needs will bear on quality. Nurse leaders should also remember that quality is a cross-departmental discipline. Quality projects often include indicators from finance, human resources, risk management, and clinical areas of the organization. These areas have bearing on quality both directly and indirectly. For example, if staffing levels are inadequate to provide timely care, patient outcomes may not be optimal. Suboptimal outcomes often lead to increased cost, so that both the patient and the organization suffer.

Most organizations have annual quality plans that bridge four different, but important, domains: regulatory requirements for quality, department-driven quality projects, clinical quality, and service quality. Each of these areas plays a vital role in ensuring the organization's performance and the outcomes for the care given to each patient.

Many hospitals use ongoing performance measurement reports. Such a report may be referred to as a dashboard or a report card. The dashboard is used to measure their organization's performance relative to a preestablished goal or plan. Dashboards can be used for financial monitoring, process measurement, or even educational competency reporting. Dashboards are effective tools because they bring together a number of important indicators in a "real time" fashion, allowing users to evaluate and adapt performance to the present, rather than after 3 or 6 months have passed. Dashboards are an effective management tool because they help to support the "check" and "act" phases of Deming's basic quality improvement cycle of plan, do, check, and act.

ISSUES IN QUALITY REPORTING

Nurse leaders, as well as organizational leadership colleagues, walk a fine line between implementing a system that is completely standardized and lacks organizational variability as well as facilitating the human factors and the art that make medicine a discipline centered on patient *care*. Many administrators find themselves caught between a patient population and care-givers who want to be able to individualize care and increase amenities and the regulators and payers who want to remove all margin of error.

Regardless of where an organization finds itself on the continuum between individualized care and complete standardization, every hospital struggles with the cost of quality improvement. Julianne Morath, COO of Children's Hospitals and Clinics of Minnesota, summarized this well at the 2008 Nursing Leadership Congress when she said, "We are asking our staff to provide 747 care in a chassis developed by the Wright Brothers."[6] Because of the vast complexity and variability within the health care system, the ability to influence and make the necessary change is a daunting responsibility. The problem is not that providers do not want to provide good care, rather, it is that it is too hard to reliably provide high-quality, safe care in such complex care environments. The federal government's current focus on process monitoring as well as outcomes is only the first step in addressing the issues of quality that are so important.

The real truth is that there is no standardized way of providing care, and not all aspects of care can be monitored in a timely or practical way. This problem is compounded by the fact that many different documentation systems exist, and as care has grown more complex, the ability of those systems to "talk" to one another has become increasingly problematic. Therefore, providers do not have an easy way to evaluate standards and their performance relative to those standards. Furthermore, the documentation process is often so laborious and cumbersome that it actually creates a barrier to good patient care. Margins of error then increase because processes are not consistently followed, and documentation is not complete. The national movement to make the switch to electronic medical records will, in time, assist in the medical record abstraction aspect of the processes being monitoring and reported. In the meantime, an enormous amount of energy will need to be applied developing expectations in reporting systems within the health care team that focus on quality and the work of the health care team because most organizations utilize manual processes to collect and assess data.

NURSE LEADERS ON THE FRONT LINES OF QUALITY

The role of the nurse leader is to help lead best practices and establish the right culture across multiple disciplines within the organization. At a minimum, the nurse leader must have the competencies necessary to design, coordinate, and advance the principles and practices for quality patient care. This can only be accomplished in collaboration with the interdisciplinary team in health care, academia, solution providers, policy makers, and the community.

At a minimum, the staff nurse and novice nurse leader must understand the role that quality plays in health care. They need to uphold the culture of quality, and they need to know that the American Nurses Association's standards of nursing professional performance state: "*Standard I. Quality of Practice: The registered nurse systematically enhances the quality and effectiveness of nursing practice.*"[7]

The nurse also must be competent in the tools for monitoring, evaluating, and reporting quality measures as well as the ability to mentor and uphold the quality processes. (Examples of tools for quality monitoring and reporting are located in the Appendix.)

WHAT IS PATIENT SAFETY?

The National Patient Safety Foundation has defined patient safety as "the avoidance, prevention, and amelioration of adverse outcomes or injuries stemming from the processes of health care."[8] Furthermore, in the IOM's book, To Err Is Human, an accident is defined as "an event that involves damage to a defined system that disrupts the ongoing or future output of that system."

For more than a decade, the nation has been focused on health care quality in response to increasing costs in care. In the mid-1990s the U.S. Department of Health and Human Services (DHHS) collected data showing that the rate of hospital deaths occurring as a result of medical errors in U.S. hospitals ranged from 2.9% in Colorado to 13.6% in New York. Aggregated across the United States, this would imply that 44,000 individuals died each year as a result of medical errors. The results from a New York study suggest the number may be as high as 98,000, making it the seventh leading cause of death in the United States.[9]

DHHS then requested that the IOM convene a committee to produce a detailed plan to reduce medical error risk by developing data standards applicable to the collection, coding, and classification of patient safety information. In June 1998, the IOM Quality of Health Care in America Committee was formed. The work of this committee resulted in the 1999 IOM report titled, *To Err Is Human: Building a Safer Healthcare System.*[10] The IOM report indicated that the annual total cost (lost income, lost household production, disability and health care costs) of preventable adverse events (medical errors resulting in injury) is estimated to be between $17 billion and $29 billion, of which health care costs represent over one half.[11]

The goal of *To Err Is Human* was to break the cycle of inaction. The status quo was not acceptable and could not be tolerated any longer. Although it was necessary for the health care system to assure the public of its efforts to provide safe care, as with any solution, there is no "silver bullet." The issue of patient safety is very complex, as are the solutions.

NURSE LEADERS INFLUENCING PATIENT SAFETY

Nursing leadership can play an integral role in assisting organizations to evaluate the "risk factors" that could have the greatest impact on improving the safety of patient care. Luckily, nurses have many tools to assist with such a review. Various health care regulatory agencies, insurers of health care organizations, advocacy groups that uphold patient safety, and patient safety consumer groups have created organizational risk assessments.

Perhaps the most prominent federal organization is the Agency for Healthcare Research and Quality (AHRQ), one of the 12 agencies within the DHHS. AHRQ's mission is to support health services research initiatives that seek to improve the quality of health care in the United States. Its goal is to improve the quality, safety, efficiency, effectiveness, and cost-effectiveness of health care for all Americans. Its broad portfolio touches on nearly every aspect of health care.[12]

Another good benchmarking and assessment tool resource comes from the Institute for Safe Medication Practices (ISMP) whose mission is "to advance patient safety worldwide by empowering the healthcare community, including consumers, to prevent medication errors."[13] Information about this tool can be found on the organization's Web site, at http://www. ismp.com

The National Quality Forum is a private, nonprofit public benefit corporation, created in 1999 in response to the need to develop and implement a national strategy for health care quality measurement and reporting. Established as a unique public-private partnership, the National Quality Forum has broad participation from more than 170 organizations that represent all sectors of the health care industry, including health care providers, consumers, employers, insurers, and other stakeholders.

Another resource is the work that has been accomplished by the Leap Frog Group. The Leap Frog Group is a voluntary program aimed at alerting the U.S. health industry through mobilizing employer purchasing power to alert them that big leaps in health care safety, quality, and customer value will be recognized and rewarded. Among other initiatives, Leap Frog works with its employer members to encourage transparency and easy access to health care information as well as rewards for hospitals that have a proven record of high-quality care.[14]

Nurse leaders will want to work with their organization's risk manager to determine which assessment tool is the right one for their organization. It may be that the organization's insurer has a recommended tool.

NURSING RESPONSE TO FACTORS INFLUENCING PATIENT SAFETY

As with quality, variability lies behind most patient safety issues. Variability in ordering and administering care contributes significantly to the risk for errors in health care. Also, as with quality, the systems involved in patient safety are deeply interrelated. Variability in one system will likely lead to variability in other systems, thereby creating nearly certain opportunity for a patient safety problem to occur. Many factors contribute to this variability, but one of the most important is communication. Many different types and layers of communication influence patient care, including discussions between the patient and provider(s), conversations between providers within the organization, and communication with providers outside the organization. The communication can be written or oral, and sometimes is simply inferred.

Improvements in patient safety have not focused on standardization of communication, largely because it would be nearly impossible to achieve. Styles of communication, education, and literacy levels, not to mention language barriers, factor into the mix. The increasing numbers of non–English-speaking patients as well as foreign-born nurses and physicians compound the opportunities for miscommunication. Furthermore, education of the various health care disciplines occurs in silos, which do not necessarily take into account the other systems at play. Silos are considered a single-discipline focused approach as opposed to a multidisciplinary team which can bring several views to the discussion. Nurse-to-nurse communication may be driven by the kardex or the patient care plan, whereas therapy professionals may communicate using a separate therapy communication tool. Physicians communicate through progress notes, which may or may not correlate with the other communication systems in use. Leaving aside the various documentation and care planning "languages" in use, there are also very real issues involving in-person communication.

Twenty years ago, the bulk of communication about a patient's care was done in real time, with the patient in the room. While it is true that technology has expanded our capacity to capture and share information, the changing ways in which we collect and relay that information has a significant downside. We no longer interface with the patient and other professionals in ways that can help us to see the whole picture.

Take, for example, a common surgical case. When a cholecystectomy was performed as a major surgical procedure and the patient stayed 5 days, we had the opportunity to talk with the patient in a more relaxed fashion, gather information, and share information with each other over multiple intersections of care. Because cholecystectomies are now primarily performed as laparoscopic procedures, our opportunities to converse with the patient, capture and document information, observe him or her, and connect with peers to plan and provide care has gone from 5 days to 5 hours, or less. The "systems" that surround caring for the patient have not changed at the pace that the advanced technology has changed.

Nursing assessment, teaching, and postoperative care still need to be performed, but in different ways. The nursing assessment is being performed over the phone several days in advance of the scheduled procedure. Nursing assessment skills must be keen in the event the information provided leads to further necessary evaluation of the patient prior to surgery. From an administrative standpoint, delays in surgery are very costly as are unexpected clinical issues. Therefore, the phone assessment, follow-up documentation, and communication with the rest of the team are all very important parts of the process.

Even when communication is clear, variability in care processes can lead to confusion and frustration. Consider the nurse who, as the coordinator of care, is responsible for collating the necessary information for ongoing patient care. If that nurse has a case load of five patients per shift, and each patient has the same diagnosis but different physicians, there is a strong likelihood of variation in each patient's order set for care. Therefore, each patient would have unique laboratory tests that must be performed, unique therapies, unique medication orders, unique patient education programs, and the list goes on. As lengths of stay continue to decrease, there is constant turnover of patients for whom this care must be coordinated, leading to increased opportunities for errors to occur. It is no wonder that, at the end of the day, the staff goes home frustrated and worried that they may have missed something in caring for their patients.

Nursing plays a key role in participating in the care regimens for patients. Little, if any, attention to this arena occurs in undergraduate education; therefore, nurses begin their careers providing care based on the physician's "pen." However, busy physicians and nurses facing increasing acuity and shorter lengths of stay may find themselves dealing with large gaps in communication when what they meant to say (and assumed the others do understand) was not explicitly said. Miscommunication and incomplete communication lead to frustration for all concerned, errors, and poor patient outcomes. Therefore, to improve communication among professionals (and with the patient), it is important to utilize multidisciplinary team planning. Although this skill is taught in most training programs, it is not consistently used in practice. Nurse leaders can help to improve safety by encouraging and supporting multidisciplinary team-based planning and communication.

Several collaborative care models exist and ought to be central to all clinical education tracks. Instead of education being provided in silos, academia needs to become proactive in developing curricula and collaborative care models that contribute to decreased variability, optimal communication, and positive patient outcomes. In the meantime, nurse leaders can work within their teams to increase multidisciplinary communication that fosters collaboration in patient care.

Instead of supporting coordinated, consistent, high-quality care, our current systems seem to reinforce erratic, uncoordinated, and confusing patient care. Again, this is a function of the multiple and varied systems that help to manage our highly complex care practices. Every nurse, and every nurse leader, wants to provide a safe, consistent environment for care. Over the past few years, use of the SBAR tool (situation, background, assessment, and recommendation) has helped to bridge some of this gap. (SBAR was a communication model originally used by the U.S. Navy nuclear submarines. The "R" in SBAR was revised for health care to indicate "recommendation" rather than "resolution," as in the original Navy model.)

SBAR guides staff in the best way to communicate a large amount of information in a succinct way when a patient's situation is escalating. It can also be used during *all* types of hand-off communication between and among providers. It is designed to improve both the manner in which information is communicated and how it is received. SBAR establishes a specific protocol to remind nurses and ancillary staff of what to assess, and how to communicate that information quickly and effectively to physicians.

The nurse initiates SBAR by assessing the situation and providing a concise statement of the problem or situation, including information such as vital signs. The nurse then provides background on what has happened, which may include mental status, physical changes, or ongoing support measures, such as the fact that the patient is receiving oxygen. Next, the nurse provides a quick assessment of what he or she assumes the problem to be. Finally, the nurse makes a recommendation to the physician, such as requesting that the physician see the patient, make a transfer, or order any necessary tests.

SBAR is also a specific tool that assists in communicating to ancillary personnel, it is a valuable component considering the large numbers of patients who are transported for testing and other diagnostic services. It provides a structure for unit-to-unit communication, such as whether a patient just received pain medication or whether an important drug regimen needs to occur during the time the patient is away form the unit.

Documentation within the patient care record is another common source of miscommunication. AHRQ recognized that the most common root causes of medical errors fell into eight categories:

1. Communication problems
2. Inadequate information flow (timeliness of critical test results, critical information for prescribing practices)
3. Human problems

4. Patient-related issues (improper patient identification, incomplete assessment, lack of a consent, etc.)
5. Organizational transfer of knowledge (lack of training and education)
6. Staffing patterns (inadequate staffing, lack of supervision)
7. Technical failures (equipment failure, implant or graft failure)
8. Inadequate policies for providing care

Improving documentation within the patient care record is a primary way to decrease confusion and potential for error. For instance, certain common abbreviations may have more than one meaning. In May 2005, the Joint Commission on Accreditation of Healthcare Organizations approved its official "Do Not Use" list, which applies (at a minimum) to all orders and all medication-related documentation that is handwritten, including free-text computer entry or orders on preprinted forms. The "Do Not Use" list includes the requirement to write out the word "unit" rather than using the abbreviation "U," and to write out "daily" or "every other day" rather than using "qd" or "qod." Similarly, providers are instructed to write out drug names such as magnesium sulfate or morphine sulfate rather than using an abbreviation such as "MS," and to write out the words "greater than" or "less than" rather than using the symbols "<" or ">." These examples emphasize how improving the accuracy of documentation contributes to the care of the patient.

Another significant factor in patient care errors is constrained time. Time can relate to the care requirements of the assigned patients as well as the nonclinical but still vital tasks related to patient care. For example, if several pages of orders are written and the nurse starts to implement and organize the plan of care to perform these orders, and then the physician cancels or significantly revises the order, this interruption in processes contributes to the time required to care for an assigned patient care group. Assignments are based on patient acuity averages and average volumes; however, the average day hardly ever reflects such average patient care needs. Nurses can expect that interruptions will occur and that they will have to change gears often in the course of their day. This, in turn, can lead to shortcuts, rushed processes, and less-than-optimal care. Balancing clinical care with the business that surrounds care is always difficult. Nurse leaders must always weigh staffing needs in order to minimize overtime while ensuring adequate resources for patient care demands.

HOW NURSE LEADERS INFLUENCE PATIENT SAFETY

In addition to encouraging multidisciplinary communication and teams, nurse leaders can help support the development of standing order sets as a means of decreasing variation and increasing safety. Helping providers to streamline their preferences in order to ensure effective use of staffing material resources is a key function of the nurse leader's role.

Nurse leaders also influence patient safety by encouraging the nursing team to advocate for patients. Occasionally, issues arise as a result of situations in which the physician and nurse disagree on a particular aspect of a patient's care plan. Nursing leadership has the opportunity and responsibility to create a culture that encourages the use of evidence-based practice and open dialogue about updates in care protocols. Further, nursing and medical staff policies need to ensure a blame-free work environment in which professionals can identify and report issues as they arise. Whether noting a process error, an impaired colleague, or even a suspected case of abuse, nurses must have the opportunity to report such issues without fear of retribution.

Finally, nursing leadership can influence patient safety by helping to create an environment that encourages and supports patients becoming their own best advocates. Through bedside interaction and patient and caregiver education, nurses and their leaders can help all participants in the care process decrease variation, improve structure and process standardization, and strive for best-in-class care.

> *"Over the next 10 years nurses and nursing leadership will be judged as to whether patients are safer and better outcomes are achieved. As leaders we must collaborate with those who serve the patient and balance imperatives that surround the delivery of health care."*
>
> —Judith K. Walker, MS, RN, NEA-BC, PLNC;
> Past President,
> AONE Council of Nurse Managers,
> Firestone, Colorado

CASE STUDY

Norma, RN, is the charge nurse on a 16-bed pediatric unit. The most frequent medical diagnosis among patients on the unit is respiratory syncytial virus (RSV). A total of 27 medical staff members have privileges to care for this population of patients. The medical staff includes neonatology, pediatric cardiology, general pediatrics, family medicine, pediatric pulmonology, trauma surgeons, and family medicine residents.

On one particular day, Norma, observed great variation in the ordering practices of the physicians caring for this patient group. There were six patients in the unit, all diagnosed with RSV. Norma was a "curious" nurse and took it upon herself to monitor and evaluate a handful of indicators for these six patients. Her findings included several different medications, lengths of stay ranging from 2 to 8 days, and various respiratory care protocols. At the same time, two different parents expressed to her that "my child is being treated differently than the one in the other room" and asked, "why is that so?"

Norma's curiosity led her to ask her supervisor whether there was an opportunity to further study this situation and evaluate a more collaborative method of delivering care to this patient population. Subsequently, the pediatric supervisor and Norma, met with the chief of the pediatric service, Dr. Kopp. Dr. Kopp acknowledged that variability existed in physician practices and suggested they all come to the table to evaluate opportunities to reduce variation. Also invited to participate were a pulmonary specialist, a case manager, and a respiratory therapist. Together this team developed a multidisciplinary practice guideline for the identified patient population.

Assessment Questions

1. How does practice variability affect staff caring for the patient, the organization's financial viability, patient and family satisfaction, and clinical outcomes?
2. What role can nursing play in recognizing symptoms of practice variability?
3. What impact does variability have on patient safety measures?
4. What key competencies are necessary in order to evaluate variability, outcomes, and improvements in patient care?
5. Why is the role of leadership important in this situation?

Best Practice

- Be able to recognize variability.
- Communication and data are key in addressing this situation.
- Medical staff leadership and nursing leadership are key in providing an environment for collaborative practice that is evidence based and multidisciplinary.
- Academia must recognize the value of teams for teaching because in the "real world," that is how care is provided and practiced.
- Ensuring clear communication is vital to quality and patient safety.
- Nurse leaders can help by constantly monitoring structures and processes in order to minimize variations in outcomes.
- Academic as well as continuing education can assist in skill and competency development in this area.

REFERENCES

1. Joint Commission on Accreditation of Healthcare Organizations. (1992). *Striving toward improvement: Six hospitals in search of quality*. Washington, DC: JCAHO.
2. Straker, David, "What is Quantity." Available at: http://sygue.com/articles/ what-is-quality/what-is-quality-4.htm
3. New York Times, December 7, 2008. Available at: http:// nytimes.com/2008/12/08/business/8hospital.htm? pagewanted=3&_1=1
4. ANA Nursing World. Available at: http://www.nursingworld.org
5. Jiang, H. J., Lockee C., Bass K., & Fraser, I. (2008). Board engagement in quality: Findings of a survey of hospital and system leaders. *Journal of Healthcare Management, 53,* 121–135.
6. 2008 Nursing Leadership Congress, Driving Patient Safety Through Transformation; Transformational Leadership: achieving the Tipping Point. Julie Morath, RN, MS, Chief Operating Officer and Vice President of Care Delivery, Children's Hospitals and Clinics Minneapolis-St. Paul, Minnesota.
7. Ballard, K. A., Arbogasat, D., Boeckman, J., et al., & American Nurses Association. (2004). *Nursing: scope and standards of practice*. Silver Spring, MD: American Nurses Association.
8. "Agenda for Research and Development in Patient Safety," National Patient Safety Foundation at the AMA. (1999, May 24). http://www.ama-assn.org/med-sci/npsf/research/research.htm
9. Centers for Disease Control and Prevention (National Center for Health Statistics). (1999). Deaths: Final data for 1997. *National Vital Statistics Reports, 47,* 19–27.
10. Institute of Medicine (1999). *To err is human: Building a better healthcare system.* Washington, DC: National Academy Press. Summary available online at: http://www.nap.edu/books/0309068371/html/
11. Thomas, E. J., Studdert, D. M., Newhouse, J., et al. (1999). Cost of medical injuries in Utah and Colorado. *Inquiry, 36,* 255–264.
12. Agency for Healthcare Research and Quality. (November 2007). *AHRQ strategic plan.* Rockville, MD: AHRQ. Available at: http://www.ahrq.gov/about/stratpln.htm
13. Institute for Safe Medication Practices. Available at: http://ismp.com
14. The Leap Frog Group. Available at: http://www.leapfrog.com

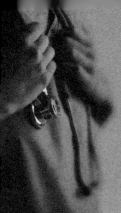

Chapter 4

HEALTH CARE POLICY

"Health care is on the cusp of standardization like never before. Public accountability and transparency will require that high quality and low costs become the focus of health care. This strategy will cause even greater streamlining, less duplication, more communication and collaboration among payers, providers, and the public."

— Pat Conway-Morana, MAd, RNC,
NEA-BC, CPHQ, FACHE;
Chief Nurse Executive,
Inova Fairfax Hospital Campus,
Falls Church, Virginia,
AONE Board of Directors

THE NATIONAL LEVEL

The U.S. health care system is very complex. The policies that surround health care add to its complexity by describing and monitoring who receives care, when care is given, and how care is rendered. The term "policy" relates to every regulation, law, and organizational rule for health care, from the unit and department level of the local hospital all the way to federal and international levels. Health care policies may pertain to clinical processes, quality and safety, financing, and ethical matters.

Nurses play an integral role in the development and implementation of health care policy. The nurse's clinical and managerial roles provide the context within which many policies are developed, reported, reviewed, and revised. Thus, for the health care leader, minimum competencies in health care policy are a must. Owing to the rapid and profound change that is occurring in health care today, the nurse leader has the responsibility to understand the broad political dynamics that have been a part of the U.S. health care system. Nursing leadership plays a significant role in recognizing and responding to the economic complexity of the system and the interactions between the key players in health care financing, and policy makers. Leaders must also recognize the roles that the culture and philosophy of the current health care system play within policy matters. For example, 20 years ago, it was very common for patients to be housed in wards or double rooms. Current cultural preferences, as well as rules regarding patient privacy, have led many organizations to convert all of their inpatient units to single rooms. Before making that change, however, hospital leaders needed to understand how single rooms would change both the cost and process of patient care. Everything from how hospitals are constructed to how patient observation is carried out has changed, and leaders have had to make policies that would accommodate those changes.

Beyond the cultural and philosophical issues affecting policy, changes in community demographics, as well as technology, safety, staffing, and patient care evolution, all drive the issues facing government regulators, health care providers, policy makers, and the consumer. As another example of how this plays out, consider how emergency departments have evolved over the years. The emergency department used to be a single room in a hospital where patients went in critical situations. That room was staffed by nurses and community physicians who "took call" for their colleagues until the patient's own physician could attend the patient. Now, however, the emergency department is a full department, acting as the primary source of hospital admissions and staffed by dedicated physicians and nurses with specialized training in emergency medicine. Their goal is to treat and release every patient who does not require admission, and they are under significant clinical and financial scrutiny to minimize lengths of stay for both emergent and observational patients. Prehospital care has shifted, too, and many emergency medical service providers are now asked to provide care to the patient so that his or her transport to the hospital is not required at all! Given recent trends by uninsured and underinsured patients to use the emergency department as their primary site of care, hospitals and their communities are changing their policies and approaches to primary and urgent care. As the changes in emergency care have evolved, so, too, have the policies that surround this type of care.

Beyond the local health care system, we are also seeing shifts in health care policy as health care becomes more globalized and patients gain the ability to access care in other regions, countries, and continents. For the first time, insurers have to consider medical tourism benefits for patients who travel to other countries for faster and cheaper access to care. Health care providers are considering the implications of telemedicine and the prospect of providing virtual consultations to patient via audiovisual linkages that span thousands of miles.

None of these evolutions comes without significant impact on both the policy and cost of care. We know that the health care system has been steadily consuming a rising proportion of national resources. In December 2008, the U.S. Congressional Budget Office (CBO) stated that information technology (IT) is the most cost-effective approach to health care reform. The CBO analyzed 115 health care proposals, including plans to expand health insurance coverage and curb health care spending. Although it did not endorse any specific option, the CBO report noted that without federal action, health costs will continue to rise and that the number of uninsured Americans will increase by nearly 1 million annually, reaching 54 million people in 2019. The report also predicted that health care spending would increase to 25% of the gross domestic product in 2025, up from 16% in 2007.[1]

According to the CBO report, a requirement for physicians and hospitals to use health IT as a condition of participating in Medicare could save the federal government $7 billion in the first 5 years and a total of $34 billion over 10 years. The savings would result from a reduction in medical errors and unnecessary tests and procedures, according to the budget office. CBO added that the health IT requirement also would lower private-sector health insurance premiums. Making those changes, however, implies a significant adaptation of patient care clinical practice, as well as documentation and billing practices. None of those changes can happen overnight or without very real modification of individual and organizational behavior. Thus, while many policies begin with a logical, well-reasoned business or social case, the implementation of those policies poses different kinds of costs—financial, behavioral, and cultural—as providers implement systems and change their practice to follow the policy.

FACTORS DRIVING HEALTH CARE UTILIZATION AND REFORM

The Aging Population

Even when providers are willing and able to make changes rapidly, the communities they serve may not be so flexible. Currently, the United States faces a rapid growth in the over-50 population. As a function of their age, older people use more health care services and require a greater complexity of care than younger people do. In some ways, older people have adapted well to technology and changes in patient care; those over 60 are increasingly Internet-savvy and health care literate. They are also fairly willing to embrace pharmaceutical interventions over surgical treatments. However, they may not be as comfortable with physician use of computers in the examination room. Nor are they comfortable with the increasing amount of documentation that their health care requires.

Nevertheless, the aging population is having a significant bearing on health care's evolving policy. The aging and retirement of the baby boomers, inflation resulting from a lack of labor (especially skilled labor) to support growing patient volumes, and the increasing pressure of government expense obligations all threaten to place a heavier burden on taxpayers, increase the cost of living, and increase sales pressure on investment markets. These factors are currently being set in motion by the aging U.S. population.

The biggest population segment in the United States is the baby boomer generation—individuals born between 1945 and 1961. (Some analysts extend the definition of baby boomer to encompass those born up through 1963.) The baby boomers account for approximately 28% of the entire U.S. population. More importantly, according to the U.S. Census Bureau, baby boomers control nearly half the nation's wealth. Right now, they are in their peak earning years and preparing for retirement. Beginning in 2010, the first baby boomers will reach age 65. Over the ensuing 15 years, that fact, coupled with existing numbers of pre-boomer retirees and a declining death rate, will result in one sixth—nearly 17%—of the population being retired, a situation that has never occurred in the history of the United States.

From the time they were born, baby boomers have created trends. As children, baby boomers were behind the explosion of Barbies, hula hoops, and primary schools. During their tenure as teenagers and young adults, automobiles and rock 'n' roll showed a similar pattern, and university enrollment reached unprecedented heights. As working adults, baby boomers have led huge expansions in housing and technology and by their sheer numbers created their very own baby boomlet generation. As we prepare for the next decade, when these boomers will begin to retire en masse, we must be cognizant not only of the effects on health care, as boomers flood emergency rooms, physician's offices, and hospitals, but also of the effects on employment, investment markets, residential real estate prices, and political decisions that will ensue over the following 25 years.[2]

Health Care Financing and the Growing Uninsured Population

Factoring in costs borne by government, the private sector, and individuals, the United States spends over $1.9 trillion annually on health care expenses, more than any other industrialized country. Researchers at Johns Hopkins Medical School estimate the United States spends 44% more per capita than Switzerland, the country with the second highest expenditures, and 134% more than the median for member states of the Organization for Economic Co-operation and Development (OECD). These costs prompt fears that an increasing number of U.S. businesses will outsource jobs overseas or shift business operations entirely offshore. U.S. economic woes have heightened the burden of health care costs on both individuals and businesses. Our competitive disadvantage is that employer-funded coverage is the structural mainstay of the U.S. health insurance system. According to the U.S. Bureau of Labor Statistics, about 71% of private employees in the United States had access to employer-sponsored health plans in 2006. A November 2008 Kaiser Foundation report notes that access to employer-sponsored health insurance has been on the decline among low-income workers, and health premiums for workers have risen 14% in the last decade. Small businesses are less likely than large employers to be able to provide health insurance as a benefit. At 12%, health care is the most expensive benefit paid by U.S. employers, according to the U.S. Chamber of Commerce.

It is difficult to quantify the precise effect high health care costs have had so far on the overall U.S. job market. Health care is one of several factors—entrenched union contracts are another—that make doing business in the United States expensive, and it is difficult to parse the effects of each factor. Moreover, economists disagree on the number of U.S. jobs that have been lost to offshoring (the transfer of business operations across national boundaries to friendlier operating environments). It is clear, however, that health care expenses affect every level of U.S. industry.

In January 2009, the human resources consulting firm Watson Wyatt predicted a further increase in health care costs of 10.6% in this year alone. As a result of the continuing increases in health care costs, employees are either going without care or self-rationing. In 2008, Watson Wyatt estimated that 17% of Americans skipped a recommended physician visit and another 17% skipped a prescription refill, while 20% of Americans have reduced retirement contributions due to health care costs. Obviously, these actions, while containing costs in the present, have the potential to drive costs the longer patients go without care. Further, as the number of unemployed people rises, the rate of those without insurance rises too. The Commonwealth Fund estimates that fewer than 10% of laid off workers elect COBRA coverage when it is offered, largely due to cost.[3] Further, because only 38% of low-wage earners are eligible for COBRA, the number of those electing such coverage is relatively small.

President Obama and Congress are working to create some stop-gap measures to help offset the issue, including continuation and expansion of the State Children's Health Insurance Program (SCHIP) and expanded Medicaid eligibility. These efforts have an element of mixed blessings: while they increase funding and make care more accessible, the cost will ultimately be borne by taxpayers, who are also bearing increased health care costs of their own. Because neither Medicare nor Medicaid covers the cost associated with care, most hospitals make up the deficit in their pricing of commercial insurance services. Recent research by Milliman indicates that the average American family of four pays $1788 more in per year health care premiums than they would if CMS reimbursement covered provider costs. This phenomenon has been dubbed the "hidden tax" by Milliman.[4]

Taken together, these factors force hospitals to compete for more preferable reimbursement rates, higher acuity patients, and more complex cases. Those who study the health care industry, including university faculty Michael Porter and Elizabeth Olmstead Teisberg, conclude that policy makers and providers have lost sight of what is really important. Teisberg writes:

> Competition is too broad because much of the competition now takes place at the level of health plans, networks, hospital groups, physician groups, and clinics. It should occur in addressing particular medical conditions. Competition is too narrow because it now takes place at the level of discrete interventions or services. It should take place for addressing medical conditions over the full cycle of care, including monitoring and prevention, diagnosis, treatment, and the ongoing management of the condition.[5]

Teisberg also said part of the reason for this disconnect is that companies have traditionally focused their attention strictly on direct costs rather than on the root cause of the costs: poor health. Teisberg cites internal corporate reports that estimate the combined costs of these additional expenses to be two-and-a-half to three times higher than the direct costs of coverage.

Clinical and Information Technology

Like most policy researchers, Porter and Teisberg acknowledge both the potential and the cost of using technology to reform our health care system. Teisberg points to the example of imaging that can be used to detect warning signs in people at risk for stroke. Imaging is expensive and thus rarely implemented as a preventive measure. However, strokes are the leading cause of long-term disability in the United States—and account for an extraordinary cost burden on the system that could potentially be reduced through the smaller, if still significant, up-front cost of imaging.

Technology can play an important role in minimizing overall health costs by making systems more efficient and decreasing the likelihood of mistakes. Jeffrey Rideout, MD, the medical director for Cisco, one of the industry's leading edge vendors of health care IT solutions, points out that U.S. health care IT spending lags behind the amounts spent by other countries on health care IT as well as what other domestic industries spend on IT. Rideout says the average company outside the health industry spends seven times as much as U.S. health care companies on IT, and companies in some wealthier industries such as banking spend up to 20 times as much. U.S. competitors abroad have also consistently outspent the U.S. government on health care IT investment. Rideout says the U.S. government invests 43 cents annually per capita on IT. The Canadian government, by contrast, spends $31 per capita.[6]

One of the most commonly cited goals of expanded IT investment is the shift to electronic medical records. Although critics worry about privacy, digitizing patient records achieves a number of goals at once. Electronic records reduce filing and storage costs and they also reduce the likelihood of errors in prescriptions and in data transfer between sites of care—flaws that can cause medical errors and prompt the need for expensive ongoing care.

Changing Federal Leadership

Some analysts believe health care reform and a weakening economy are on a collision course. Most lawmakers have come to recognize that the need for health care reform must be addressed. However, some experts worry that reform may be derailed over differences in how to accomplish it—and how much to spend. Estimates for President Obama's plan range from $634 billion or more in government spending annually over the next decade. One of the biggest sticking points will be whether to mandate that all Americans must have health care coverage, and all employers must provide coverage as a benefit. A health care reform proposal by Senator Max Baucus (D-Mont.), who heads the Senate Finance Committee, notes that:

> Despite widespread agreement on the need for reform, the task remains difficult because Americans do not necessarily agree on how to achieve it. Although a majority of respondents would support a mandate on employers to provide coverage, a "Medicare-for-all" single-payer option, or a mandate that all individuals purchase coverage, opposition to each of these options is also somewhat substantial.[7]

WHAT CAN THE NURSE AND NURSE LEADER DO?

Within the operations of the day-to-day health care environment, health care policy is often overlooked. Numerous bylaws, policies, regulations, licensing requirements, and mission/vision and value statements exist for every organization. It would be difficult if not impossible to know each of these policies in detail; however, all nurse leaders are responsible for knowing both that these policies exist and their potential organizational and clinical implications.

Step One: Familiarize yourself with the work of your professional organization. Professional organizations help nurse leaders by identifying, reviewing, and advocating for policies of interest to nursing practice. Specialty organizations can also help to advise and assist members in their implementation of policies through member alerts, continuing education courses, and member forums. It is worthwhile to remember that the professional organizations also have policies of their own that pertain to the respective organization's mission and position on key areas of interest. As a nurse leader, it is important to participate in your professional association so that you have access to the latest information as it may relate to your duties and responsibilities.

Step Two: Familiarize yourself with the policies of your organization and the nursing department. The framework surrounding health care policy within an organization is provided by the organizational and corporate bylaws that denote the purpose and function of the organization. Within the bylaws the name of the corporation is noted along with various organizational directives and objectives. Of even greater value is the policy information, often called "rules and regulations," that describes the intent of the bylaws. In nursing governance, bylaws, rules, and regulations exist that may include a plan for nursing care within the nurse leader's facility. Components of the plan vary among facilities and may include the definition of nursing, the nursing division's vision/value statement and philosophy, as well as the delivery model, staffing plan, applications of nursing standards, and possibly utilization of shared governance.

NURSE LEADERS, POLICY DEVELOPMENT, AND GOVERNANCE

The governing bylaws as well as policies and procedures provide the framework within which the individual sections of the organization operate. Whether these sections are organized according to service lines, product lines, or departments such as nursing or radiology, their nurse leaders are involved with, and often directly responsible for the development of and compliance with policies, standards of practice, and organizational bylaws that influence the overall organization.

In 1981, Tim Porter-O'Grady, PhD, developed a concept of shared decision making referred to as "shared governance."[8] Shared governance is defined as a systematic means of providing a communication forum for nursing that effects individual input into the professional practice of nursing. Current governance models make use of this concept to varying degrees, depending on the organization and the cultural readiness of the organization to uphold the model.

A key element of shared governance is the presence of nursing-driven councils that have primary responsibilities for such things as education, practice, leadership, research, quality, and advanced practice. The Magnet Recognition Program® recognizes that organizations that achieve such recognition are generally flat (non-hierarchical), flexible, and decentralized. In these high-performing organizations, nurses throughout the organization are involved in self-governance and in decision-making processes that establish standards of practice and address issues of concern. The flow of information becomes bidirectional in that it flows "in and out as well as among" staff, leadership, and others who contribute to the patient care processes. Shared leadership approaches take various forms, which mature and evolve over time. The philosophy and its embracement by leadership and staff become the underpinnings of the success of this governance model.

Most often, the shared leadership "groups" that are formed are referred to as "councils." The councils meet on a regular basis and then the chairs of these councils also meet in a sort of "cabinet meeting" to share their activities and work on cross-council (bidirectional function) activities. The cabinet allows the practice council to know what the education council is doing, as well as what the leadership council is engaged in, and vice versa.

Shared governance is one means by which to become involved in health care policy at the individual and organizational level. Many staff nurses who aspire to leadership positions may see council involvement as a first step on that journey. Staff is encouraged to participate in the shared governance system so that the empowerment message is heard throughout the organization. For example, an organization might have an interest in the role and reimbursement of the advanced practice nurse. The advanced practice council could then study the regulatory information and provide feedback to both the nursing division and the organization overall. This one action could have profound effects on a singular discipline within the organization. This example also highlights how nurses and their colleagues can participate in the process by which an organization's policy evolves.

Such cross-organizational involvement allows nursing leadership to incorporate many perspectives in the positions and activities for which they advocate organization-wide. Various models exist to depict communication and collaboration between and among professional colleagues. A popular shared leadership model is depicted in a circular fashion (Fig. 4–1). A legislative/hierarchical model is also widely used and functional (Fig. 4–2).

We often hear the phrases "grassroots effort," "your vote counts," and "as an individual, you can make a difference" in the context of political campaigns. Whether at the bedside or sitting in a professional organization meeting, nurses have the opportunity (and responsibility) to work on policy issues. Keep in mind that every policy has some influence—direct or indirect—on patient care. Therefore, nurses should be aware of medical staff bylaws and policies as well as the rest of the organization's policies. Nurses and nurse leaders, especially should be sensitive to those times when staff may be tempted to do a "work around" rather than comply with a particular policy. The term "work around" depicts a shortcut performed in response to various factors, such as complexity of the designed process or the fact that the designed process takes longer than the provider desires. Enough literature exists to acknowledge

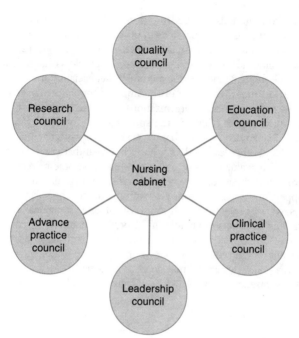

Figure 4–1   Typical shared governance model.

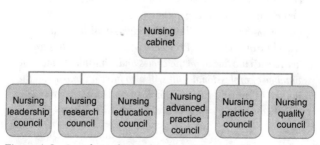

Figure 4–2   Legislative/hierarchical model.

that work arounds can lead to errors and greater patient safety risks, as well as additional steps in the work process. When these work arounds are known, it behooves everyone in the organization to examine the policy, identify the respective problems that encourage the shortcut, and develop a mutually beneficial solution.

At all times, the voice of the nurse is the voice that helps improve patient care. Organizations often recognize the chief executive officer (CEO) as the spokesperson for the organization. Remember, though, that nurses have a perspective that the CEO and other leaders do not have. It is vital that everyone recognize the value of his or her own role and become involved in improving these complex systems. When an organization offers opportunities to learn more, get involved. Identify the policy makers, whether they work with your hospital, or with regional, state, or federal leaders. Your role in advocacy is a means to ensure needs for today as well as for tomorrow. As an advocate for your patients and a provider of care, your voice is an important piece of the policy puzzle and may go far to influence the development of organizational, state, and federal legislation and policy.

"Rural health care will be drastically changed because of the demographics within these populations. Many of the communities in rural states that have a hospital or nursing home will not have a population large enough to support one or both of the facilities. Residents will be required to travel farther for care. Providers will not be able to provide 'outreach' care due to inefficiencies and windshield time. The number of professional staff will also have an impact on the ability to provide care. Technology will need to provide a significant role for future rural health care delivery."

—Terry Watne, MS, RN; Administrative Director, Altru Health System, Grand Forks, North Dakota

CASE STUDY

One in nine people has chronic kidney disease.[9] The number of people diagnosed with chronic kidney disease rose 30% in the past decade, and it now accounts for 24% of Medicare's overall spending.[9] Furthermore, the incidence of kidney disease continues to rise sharply, increasing 3.4% between 2005 and 2006, alone. Medicare provides funding for chronic kidney disease through its end stage renal disease (ESRD) program. In 2008, ESRD patients accounted for 1% of Medicare beneficiaries and 7% of total Medicare spending. Total spending for ESRD (Medicare and other payers included) is now $33.6 billion per year. One might wonder how this example relates to policy.

Karen has been passionate about the renal population since she began working as a staff nurse in the dialysis unit in 1976. Since that time, Karen has taken it upon herself to become familiar with the rules of, and participate in, the renal network that oversees care for patients with ESRD in defined areas of the United States. The renal network was established by Medicare to monitor policy, evaluate patient outcomes, and assist providers in providing the best care to this fragile patient population.

The renal network and other professional organizations for renal nurses and administrators have developed "talking points" that can be used at the local level to influence health care policy. These talking points were developed as part of a national strategy to educate the public, as well as state and federal representatives.

Most recently, the greatest issue affecting the renal population has been the risk of death from cardiovascular disease in conjunction with chronic kidney disease. The National Institutes of Health noted the importance of detecting and treating cardiovascular risk factors in patients with kidney disease.[10] Karen took it upon herself to become involved professionally as the advocacy representative for her state. Initially she met with her supervisor at her place of employment to ensure that the work she was doing was supported by her employer. Karen then met with her state senators, as well as the state's congressional representatives to discuss this growing and very expensive health care issue.

When the state and federal legislators held town hall-style meetings in her state, Karen was there with her folder and the talking points that were imperative to the financial and clinical success of this national program. It was through such grassroots efforts by many individuals that increased attention is now being paid to cardiovascular risk in chronic kidney disease patients.

 Assessment Questions

1. What is the most burning issue for you as a nurse in providing care for your patients?
2. If you could help change the impact you have on patient's lives, what change would you make?
3. How would you go about influencing this change?
4. Are you a member of your professional organization? Have you used this avenue to address your burning issue?
5. What issues locally and nationally are being discussed and how do these issues relate to your burning issue?
6. What can you do to see that your burning issue is recognized and addressed by those in charge of health care policy?

Best Practice

- Recognize issues that can be addressed in an advocacy manner for your patients and your profession.
- Engage colleagues and your immediate supervisor in affirming the issue and possibly in assisting you in determining how to "take the next steps."
- Do not be intimidated when articulating your talking points. Remember, you know more about your business than those your are speaking to and educating.
- Assess your local, state, and federal contacts.
- Always highlight the return on investment of your burning issue in terms of the cost and clinical outcomes for your patients.
- Evaluate what the burning issues are at the local, state, and federal level that may be similar to your own burning issue. Use that opportunity to bridge the issues and foster collaboration and even greater results based on the power of numbers.

REFERENCES

1. Pear, R. (2008, December 19). Budget Office Sees Hurdles in Financing Health Plans. *The New York Times.* Retrieved from http://www.newyorktimes.com
2. Renner, C. MedAmerica Financial Services newsletter. Available at: http://www.medamerica.com/mafs/Newsletters/Newsletters.asp
3. Doty, M. M., Rustgi, S. D., Schoen, C., & Collins, S. R. (2009, January). Maintaining health insurance during a recession: Likely COBRA eligibility. The Commonwealth Fund, Vol. 49. Available at:http://www.commonwealthfund.org/Content/Publications/Issue-Briefs/2009/Jan/Maintaining-Health-Insurance-During-a-Recession—Likely-COBRA-Eligibility.aspx

4. Report describes "hidden tax" resulting from public program underpayments. Available at: http://www.milliman.com/expertise/healthcare/publications/rr/pdfs/hospital-physician-cost-shift-RR12-01-08.pdf

5. Redefining Healthcare, Harvard Business School Publishing, Michael E Porter and Elizabeth Olmstad Teisberg, May 2006.

6. Anderson, G. F., Frogner, B. K., Johns, R. A., & Reinhardt, U. E. (2006). Health care spending and use of information technology in OECD countries. The Commonwealth Fund, Vol. 42. Available at: http://www.commonwealthfund.org/Content/Publications/In-the-Literature/2006/May/Health-Care-Spending-and-Use-of-Information-Technology-in-OECD-Countries.aspx

7. Baucus, M. (2009). *Call to action: Health reform 2009,* p. 17. Available at: http://finance.senate.gov/healthreform2009/finalwhitepaper.pdf

8. Porter-O'Grady, T., & Finnegan, S. (1984). *Shared governance for nursing: A creative approach to professional accountability.* Rockville, MD: Aspen Publishers.

9. The Facts About Chronic Kidney Disease. Available at: http://www.kidney.org/kidneydisease/.Retrieved July 18, 2009.

10. National Institutes of Health press release, October, 8, 2008. Available at: http://www.nih.gov/news/health/oct2008/niddk-08.htm. Retrieved July 18, 2009.

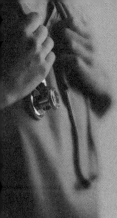

Chapter 5
TECHNOLOGY

"Technology will become the most profound next step in health care reform. The ability to utilize technology for patient care management will serve to enhance the quality, safety, and efficiency in our health care system."

—Donna Herrin, MSN, RN, NEA-BC, FACHE;
Clinical Associate Professor,
University of Alabama,
Huntsville, Alabama;
Senior Advisor, Methodist Healthcare, Memphis,
Tennesse;
2009 President, AONE Board of Directors

WHAT IS HEALTH CARE TECHNOLOGY?

Technology is both a vital and an ever-changing element in health care. Technology has multiple roles in an organization—everything from marketing and communications via the organization's Web site to clinical documentation and support, to patient safety, to operational logistics, coding, and billing. As quickly as the types and formats of technology evolve, the library of opinion about how that technology should be used to improve health care grows faster. Within this chapter we will review the role of technology and the many ways in which nurse leaders can leverage technology for improved efficiency and productivity in patient care. It is important to note that technology is a tool to leverage existing work processes and should not be considered an end in itself.

First, we begin with an overview of how technology has evolved. Health care technology has made significant strides over the past 25 years, and the future will hold even faster rates of innovation and expansion. The following list provides a brief historical review:

- **1960s and early 1970s**—Medicare and uniform billing practices are introduced, and use of telephones for internal and external communications expands.
- **1970s**—Advances are made in diagnostic technology, with minimal associated clinical technology advancements. The use of television as an educational medium expands.

  The first iterations of computerized scheduling and staffing systems are seen, as well as automation of timekeeping systems. Still, pneumatic tube systems remain the fastest way of moving information and material within hospitals.

- **1980s**—Nursing computerized documentation systems start to emerge. Early systems are primarily stand alone with little integration. Physician's offices begin to use message services, fax machines, and other means of transporting information outside of the normal administrative processes and the normal workday. The earliest forms of the Internet allow for messaging and other data warehousing (largely in academic settings). Medical libraries, following university libraries, begin automating catalogs and creating digital repositories of journals and older material.

- **1990s**—Radiological systems move from analog to digital modalities. Digital modalities provide the opportunity for a much higher quality product and the ability to enhance diagnostic work. Microsoft Windows transforms clerical and administrative functions to include a fairly universal system for word processing, spreadsheet analytics, database development, and presentation formatting. Rather than using less paper, many organizations find themselves keeping more records. Filing and documentation systems grow by a similar means. Similarly, increasing automation in supply chain and financial systems makes funds transfer and supply chain logistics faster. Integration becomes an attractive concept, though with minimal application. Clinical documentation at the bedside is relatively rare. The technology market is proposing "best of breed" for greater clinician use and applicability. Many small entrepreneurial companies emerge.

- **2000**—The focus on automation and speed from the 1990s evolves to a focus on efficiency, safety, and transparency. Legacy systems (systems and applications that have been in use for an extended period of time) find they cannot keep up with innovation, especially as Windows formats become the norm. Larger companies achieve flexibility by purchasing the smaller niche providers. Integration grows to include internal systems as well as systems across the continuum of care. Consumers are increasingly media savvy and therefore more informed and sensitive to price and quality. There is an increased willingness by hospitals to finance technology, although there is also increasing competition for technology resources across the clinical and administrative domains. Surgical robotics, telemedicine, and other clinical innovations improve standardization and specificity of clinical care. However, implementation is hampered by a significant variation in technology utilization across providers, as well as internal variation in staff and provider acceptance of the use of mobile devices—such as personal digital assistants (PDAs), laptop computers, notebooks, cell phones, and iPods—that have become the norm for both providers and patients. WebMD and health care information sites are among the most frequently accessed Web sites. There is increased use of external coding and billing, with minimal integration among the providers and systems. Nursing informatics evolves as a field unto itself.

- **2009**—Portability and interoperability are the key metrics among technology providers. Federal and state initiatives have provided momentum to increase communication to all. Examples include archiving systems, electronic health records, and physician portals for laboratory, medication management, and treatment regimens. These systems, while new and conceptual for the industry, are becoming reimbursement dependent.

Not only does technology influence health care reimbursement, it also provides for transparency. The first steps toward transparency began when the federal government provided organizations with a nominal financial incentive to participate in the submission of certain quality indicators. These incentives grew to become requirements for participating in the Medicare program. The data being submitted currently are now available publicly. Technology has enabled consumers, insurers, and providers with the means to monitor and evaluate their use (purchases) of health care products and have a far greater voice in their health care destiny. It is not uncommon for a Medicare patient to search for the "best doctor" or "best hospital" and choose to travel across the continental United States for a surgical procedure. Such transparency and consumer-driven health care will increasingly become the norm, not the exception.

In the setting of transparency, it is important that staff nurses understand their role. Nursing staff can have a significant impact on the data currently being submitted for indicators such as the following: "Did the patient receive a pneumonia vaccine prior to discharge?" "Did the patient receive the prescribed antibiotic 1 hour prior to surgery?" "How will the patient's perception of the care be scored on the opinion survey that is administered by the federal government?" All of these measures are being collected, analyzed, and reported at the federal level. These data are then utilized to determine not only the quality of patient care but also the level of reimbursement that facilities (including physicians) will receive.

Despite the explosion in information systems and technology, administrators still hear the complaint that nurses "don't have time to spend with their patients like they used to." Applied correctly, technology at the bedside enhances and provides additional time for patient care, as well as opportunities for improved communication, education, and support of the patient and family.

The key is that phrase, "applied correctly." The health care system is on the cusp of an explosion in the development and implementation of systems that provide for the longitudinal exchange of health care information while also allowing for immediacy and ease of access to information. The goal is to synthesize the data to provide better quality and safer patient care that will then lead to greater efficiency and lower cost. Getting to that point, however, will require a massive effort to coordinate and integrate a maze of complex, expensive systems that were designed at different times and with different sets of goals in mind.

FEDERAL POLICIES CHANGING THE HEALTH CARE TECHNOLOGY LANDSCAPE

As discussed in earlier chapters, the overwhelming and growing cost of health care demands that we overcome the current technology barriers in order to create a unified strategy. The February 5, 2009 edition of *Computerworld* noted:

> President Barack Obama's plan to inject $25 billion into the health care industry could create a technological divide between large and small health care organizations, according to doctors and health care professionals. And some worry that his efforts to create a national electronic health records (EHR) system could affect the quality of health care in the U.S. The Health Information Technology for Economic and Clinical Health Act or HITECH would provide roughly $25 billion for the creation of a national EHR system that would fundamentally change the health care system.[1]

Under HITECH, physicians would be eligible for between $40,000 and $65,000 if they show they are using information technology (IT) to improve the quality of care. The money that is allocated will not be used for incentives for large hospitals who have already rolled out EHRs or for those planning to roll them out. It is believed this legislation may lead to a groundswell of technology adoption for the smaller health care operations with little rhyme or reason—leading to even greater confusion among the players.

This same kind of demand has become a reality in the area of prescriptive practices. The U.S. government is piloting a number of electronic prescribing (e-prescribing) initiatives. E-prescribing allows for timely prescribing, fewer risks associated with handwritten prescriptions, increased patient safety and trending ability, as well as greater patient and provider satisfaction with the prescribing process. Recognizing that the migration to e-prescribing requires cash investment and changes in behavior, the Centers for Medicare and Medicaid Services (CMS) are piloting a project that will give providers a series of bonuses for adopting e-prescribing between 2009 and 2013.

Government support for technology was growing even before President Obama's recommended stimulus packages. The National Conference of State Legislatures indicated in late 2008 that in the previous 18 months, "more than 130 bills that contained at least some provision for health IT were enacted . . . in 44 states and the District of Columbia—triple the number enacted in the same 2005–2006 period."[2] Financing laws accounted for nearly one third of the total and were spread among 25 states. Federal and state support also promoted technology financing, e-prescribing, and regional health information exchanges.

Development of regional health care IT centers (often called regional health information organizations, or RHIOs) will help to ensure interoperability across systems and organizations. The RHIOs assist in bringing health care stakeholders together within a defined geographical area and govern the health information exchange. The U.S. Department of Defense provides a model for RHIOs whereby the records for military personnel are accessible regardless of where an individual is stationed.

THE ULTIMATE GOAL: REDUCTION IN SYSTEM VARIATION

As discussed earlier in Chapter 3, the most important hurdle to overcome in using technology is reducing variation. Although most quality concerns stem from variations in *process,* another issue with technology is a variation in *structure.* Simply put, when systems are not interoperable (they do not "talk" to each other), it creates issues for patients as well as providers. Even when organizations are technologically rich in their documentation and clinical systems, interfaces among the various clinical documentation systems and the diagnostic clinical devices may be minimal. Think about this from the patient's point of view. Most patients have multiple providers of care, doing different things at different times. A diabetic patient, for example, might have an internist, an endocrinologist, a nutritionist, a cardiologist, a physical therapist, and other care providers. Unless all of those providers are employed within the same system, there is only a slight chance that their information systems will be linked. Given the variation in practices and locations where patients receive care, it is close to impossible to reconcile all the tests, evaluations, treatments, and follow-up care that a patient receives. The patient becomes his or her own historian and risks redundancy as well as fragmentation and gaps in care.

This creates a problem for providers as well; they are likely to repeat testing and have missed communication, and may even have conflicts in treatment plans. The potential for medical errors (and frustration) are huge. Furthermore, having gone to the trouble of implementing a system designed to increase efficiency and productivity, many professionals find themselves having to do additional work simply to share information across systems.

Clearly a monumental shift in our approach to health care IT is on the horizon. For now, however, we need to be aware of how nurses approach the current technology, and how nurse leaders can improve approaches to future discussions and decision making relating to technology.

CLINICAL DOCUMENTATION SYSTEMS

Numerous software programs exist for clinical documentation, yet not all organizations use software to their advantage. Some organizations have few if any clinical documentation systems and continue to chart manually. Others use a software program, but only for certain portions of the patient care process. Many physicians still are skeptical about the value of clinical documentation for managing patient care. They see the system as purely a nursing documentation system.

For organizations that do use an electronic documentation system, there can be variation in what gets documented. Some of the systems chart by exception, others do not. Charting by exception means that the only time charting occurs is when the nursing assessment or a value is outside the acceptable norm, i.e., an "exception". If, for instance, the patient's skin was evaluated and was normal in condition, no charting would be performed. Charting by exception can provide other caregivers and members of the team a false sense of normalcy about the patient's condition unless all providers chart accurately. When using a charting-by-exception methodology, assumptions are made that the condition of the skin (or other parameter) was evaluated.

Many other documentation systems exist for ancillary departments such as dietary, respiratory care, physical therapy, and other services. Some systems may have order entry options, others may not. In this sense, automated charting systems can appear to be just as "siloed" as the paper chart.

Technology is used widely for diagnostics; however, its use for documentation, ordering, and reporting varies widely across the United States. Regardless of the system used by an organization, the goals for any clinical documentation program should be the same:

1. Effective communication infrastructure to provide efficient, effective, and equitable patient care.
2. Data flexibility for use in key areas such as disease management, public health trending, strategic service planning, and focused public and patient education outreach.

3. Creation of a lifelong patient care record that the individual can access and "travel" as needed.
4. Interoperability with supply chain, billing, and performance improvement systems.

Of the preceding goals, four areas need special attention: billing, patient safety, administrative management, and behavior change. Optimizing the use of technology involves process and behavior changes; these can and will be provided by the development and application of standards by users.

TECHNOLOGY USED IN BILLING

Remember that one of the initial drivers of health care technology was the creation of Medicare and uniform billing standards. When standardized billing codes were established, the providers realized an electronic coding and billing system would be imperative as part of the payment process. The electronic means assured greater accuracy in coding, which increased the timeliness of payment receipt. The electronic systems also created means to store, mine, and analyze practice data for better organizational planning, management, and patient care.

TECHNOLOGY USED IN PATIENT SAFETY

It was not long before the approaches to documentation and analysis for financial data spread to the quality and patient safety arenas. Technology drives patient care before, during, and after the hospital stay. Before the patient arrives at the hospital, technology systems help model the level of staffing, equipment, and resources that a patient might need while at the hospital. Communication systems help prehospital emergency care providers and physician offices relay information about the patient to the hospital clinical and records staff. During the hospital stay, electronic clinical information systems, telemetry, and myriad diagnostic technologies help assess, monitor, and document patient status and care. After the patient is discharged, technology helps clinical staff assess the safety, timeliness, effectiveness, and efficiency of care.

Specific to safety, technology drives items such as fall monitors, medication dispensing systems, bar coding of instruments, pharmaceuticals, and specialized patient mattresses. Each of these items is designed to ensure that patients do not experience unnecessary dangers posed by the resource-intense and complex care provided. Many researchers have studied the effect that technology has on patient outcomes. In addition to the specific safety items indicated above, researchers have noted that safety is an almost universal outcome when computerized medical record documentation is utilized.

In the January 26, 2009 electronic issue of *Modern Healthcare*, Joseph Conn noted, "When computers replace paper, patient mortality rates drop 15% during hospitalization, among other metrics."[3] Recounting a study done at Johns Hopkins, Mr. Conn went on to note a process whereby researchers divided hospital clinical IT systems into four categories: medical notes and records, test results, order entry, and clinical decision support. Physicians from the 41 hospitals represented in the study were asked to rank their organizations' systems across these four domains. Researchers then evaluated the relationship between the physicians' rankings of the systems and the rates of inpatient death, complications, costs, and length of stay for a cohort of more than 100,000 patients over the age of 50 admitted to the participating hospitals in 2005 and 2006. In addition to lower overall mortality rates, hospitals in the study with higher scores for computerized order-entry systems posted 55% lower odds of death for coronary artery bypass graft patients and 9% lower odds of death for patients with myocardial infarction. For direct care nursing, technology clearly serves as a powerful safety net for quality patient care. Nurse leaders must constantly assess what tools are necessary and available for professional nurses to effectively and efficiently do their job. Bar code technology in medication administration provides a great example. This safety guard provides significant assurance that the Right patient is given the Right medication, at the Right dose, at the Right time. Bar code technology, however, is not 100% fail-safe. Thus, while the nursing leadership may have identified the long-range benefit of having such technology in place, it must never replace the professional judgment of the nurse at the bedside. In the process of using the barcoding equipment, the nurse must continue to apply the standard of practice of assessing the 4 R's.

Aside from their immediate use to keep the patients safe, many of these systems (including medication dispensing systems, telemetry, and bar coding), can be used for retrospective clinical and administrative monitoring. For instance, in the study noted above, the use of computerized order entry was associated with lower average costs per admission and 16% lower odds of developing complications across all reasons for admission. Therefore, the information system serves two roles—reinforcing best practice to keep patients safe, and providing meaningful data about the outcomes of clinical and administrative outcomes of care.

Data drawn from systems used on individual units can help to populate systems across the organization. Nurse-sensitive data, such as patient fall data or infection control data, are good examples of information that can be used to assess unit-based practices as well as the practice for the entire division of nursing. The overall data provide summary information that can be used to exemplify best practices within the organization and to provide educational opportunities within and across the organization.

The data can also be used for evaluation and planning on a larger scale. With the emergence of evidence-based practice and evidence-based care, metrics from patient populations can be used to determine best practices within an organization as well as for benchmarking with others locally, regionally, and nationally. This access to data enables nurses to provide care that is more standardized and less prone to error, and to misinterpretation. The data also allows frontline nursing staff to react and make practice changes in a more timely basis.

PLANNING FOR AND IMPLEMENTING TECHNOLOGY SOLUTIONS

As information and technology systems evolve, the interrelationship between clinical documentation for patient safety and data aggregation for planning and evaluation becomes ever more involved. As organizations increase, update, and interconnect their technology systems, some very critical questions come into play. Key among these is the need to clarify goals. How will this technological innovation help to create more efficient, streamlined workflow processes? Will the technological application help to improve the current environment of care? In order to answer these questions, it is often important to map out existing processes, and to identify where gaps occur between the current state and the desired future state. Will the technology help to bridge those gaps, and how easy will it be to implement and maintain the changes in practice and behavior that the new system will require? Sample questions that a nurse leader might ask as part of an ongoing technology assessment include:

- Are bladder scanners readily available or is a "straight cath" routine for suspected urine retention?
- Are the necessary patient care equipment needs, such as intravenous poles, scales, and digital blood pressure cuffs with pulse oximetry capability, readily accessible to the patient care staff?
- Have the nurses provided adequate feedback about their needs?
- Do these supporting technological devices automatically "drop" their data into the patient record or is charting being performed manually on a "cheat sheet" and placed in the pocket of the caregiver, only later to be charted in the automated record? Does this duplication of efforts increase the chance for documentation errors?

One of the best ways to identify technology needs is by mapping current processes to identify gaps that could be improved by being made faster, more consistent, or more efficient overall.

In addition to mapping current processes and correlating them into goals, it is important to create standards of practice for the new technology. Making, and sustaining, behavioral changes is vital to ensure full and optimized technology implementation. However, behavioral changes are never easy—for individuals or groups. The standards help to articulate and measure how adoption of the technology should occur, and they should indicate the following: a clear statement of why the technology is being adopted, the advantages of using the technology, how it is to be used, who is to use it, and the repercussions if individuals do not evolve their practice to meet the standard.

THE NURSE LEADER'S MANY ROLES IN TECHNOLOGY

Despite the many advantages associated with a high-tech health care practice, the proliferation of technology can be overwhelming and intimidating to patients and nurses alike. Nurse leaders play a critical role by helping to advance patient and provider understanding of technology's value.

For example, when an organization institutes a point-of-care documentation system that is located either in or close to the patient's room, nurse leaders must establish, role model, and manage the new standard for utilization of the new system and technology. The implementation of such technology into the work environment ought to include not only a means to streamline the current manual process of documentation, but also to expect staff behavioral change. Based upon combination of written standards, education, and coaching, nurse leaders can demonstrate and articulate the reason such standards are established and why point-of-care documentation is more valuable (timely, accurate, efficient, patient centered).

The difficulty that many organizations face is determining how to address violations in policy and practice, which often happen at the outset when the new technology is introduced. Mentoring is one way to improve comfort with the new standard. Nurse leaders can help to identify those elements of the technology that are confusing or cumbersome, and can work with frontline nursing staff and the IT staff to overcome those concerns. In the context of their own use of the technology, they can help to model the organization's enthusiasm and commitment to the technology's value. Another way to increase the comfort level is to create a group approach, whereby peers evaluate the evidence-based literature and help create the clinical precedence for the new standard. This is important for two reasons:

First and foremost, nurse leaders must recognize the value that comes from empowered, proactive clinical practice review. Years ago, the "expert nurse" on the unit influenced the culture of the unit and the way in which care was delivered. Today, the literature, access to data, and best practices provide a greater opportunity to translate what expert nurses "had in their heads" and "just knew" to a broader spectrum of the nursing staff. Through the use of technology, every staff nurse and leader now has the ability to study, "know," and practice in a way that provides for optimal patient outcomes.

Second, by studying the literature, the individual nurses will gain a better understanding of the context behind the technology's development and use. When the nursing staff understand the purpose behind implementation of technology and the associated standards for its use, the level of compliance will be enhanced. As nurses witness their leaders and peers embracing the new technology, and the evidence behind it, they will use it to enhance their own practice as well as the care provided to the patients.

Furthermore, use of the evidence (and the data generated from the information systems themselves) will help nurses to uphold the use of technology in their individual and unit-based practice. In order to reach that point, however, the nurse leader must constantly acknowledge and work to positively influence the requisite changes to deeply ingrained behaviors and culture that technology can represent. Leadership plays a key role in influencing such change, through communication, role modeling, observations, coaching, rewarding of positive behavior, and disciplining when appropriate.

An example of providing rewards was the use of a "traveling" bar code trophy at St. Alexius Medical Center in Bismark, North Dakota. In 1991, when the use of bedside barcoding for supplies and medication administration was introduced and implemented, the unit with the highest level of compliance was rewarded with a traveling trophy. It became a competitive event whereby the units attempted to "keep" the traveling trophy longer than their peer units. Today, 95% of all medications are scanned in the patients' room and less than 1% of all supplies fall to "lost charges." This reward process led to changing behavior in a positive manner:

Quality and patient safety underpin the proper use of technology, and should staff choose not to follow establish standards, the use of disciplinary action may be necessary.

LEADERSHIP COMPETENCIES IN TECHNOLOGY PLANNING AND ADOPTION

Before nurse leaders or anyone in a leadership position can provide mentorship for technology adoption, they must develop their own acumen and competency in technology. All health care leaders need to have a role in the acquisition, implementation, and evaluation of technology for their organizations. Table 5–1 outlines key questions and approaches that nurse leaders might use in technology planning. This list is not all-inclusive; however, it highlights components that are critical to implementation of a successful organizational and nursing leadership IT strategy.

RESOURCE PLANNING FOR TECHNOLOGY

The two greatest barriers to implementation of technology are cultural adoption issues and cost. The challenge of overcoming the human factors in workflow process redesign and individual adoption of technology is a fluid one in which multiple factors are at play. Cost, on the other hand, is more absolute. Regardless of negotiated discounts or payment plans, implementation of any technological advance represents hard choices about budgeting and resource allocation that must have an associated measurable benefit over time. Identifying the true return on investment can be quite difficult, especially because most technology creates a period of inefficiency during the learning curve when users are

Table 5–1   Questions and Approaches in Planning for
            Technology Acquisition

Core Competencies	Planning Assessment
Knowledge of information technology (IT) industry	Obtain general industry knowledge.
Knowledge of organization's IT plan	Identify the organizational IT plan and vision and how it relates to nursing. Before acquiring new technology, obtain staff and leadership feedback on the effectiveness and gaps in current workflow processes.
Knowledge of organizational culture and readiness for change	Make site visits with staff to assess readiness and identify peer champions.
Knowledge of the potential interoperability of new and legacy systems	Play an active role in decision processes, and participate when vendors meet with the chief information officer (CIO).
Knowledge of vendor ratings with the technology	Research vendor training and support of the product. Obtain reviews from other organizations.
Knowledge of the RFP vendor request for purchase process	Focus on policy and standards development.
Knowledge of the ROI (return on investment) process	Identify and monitor measures of success, including patient safety and user satisfaction.
Legal counsel contractual review	Determine warranties, contingency plans, downtime, equipment service and upgrades, replacements, etc.
Ongoing IT strategy	Develop a collaborative evaluation process for vendor and provider stakeholders and review on a regular basis.

changing from one process to another. Electronic health records are a great example of this dynamic: although adoption of an EHR is shown to have great benefit over time, during the first year lower productivity and higher rates of redundancy are common as paper records are transferred to electronic files and users get used to navigating the new systems.

Because of the expense of technology, a great amount of diligence is required when evaluating strategy, purchasing, implementation, and evaluation. Multiple value-added factors need to be considered, including clinical, management, and administrative aspects. Furthermore, the organization needs to consider how its technology plans can be leveraged on a regional level. For instance, if a single hospital implements a particular clinical documentation system, will it allow for greater interoperability with other providers and payers? If so, that may help to mitigate the cost of its implementation.

Other considerations are the likely life cycle of the product and its continuing operating costs. Licenses and supplies are key items to consider here. When assessing various systems, the tool itself is very important. However, a complete evaluation that includes ongoing licensing, human resources, and other "invisible" resources must be a part of the purchase and implementation plan; otherwise acquisition and implementation of the new technology is doomed to fail.

It is also important to keep in mind how applicable the potential technology will be to the population being served. Take diagnostic imaging as an example. Many community hospitals feel they need to invest in highly sensitive imaging equipment in order to stay competitive. However, the investment in a 64-slice computed tomography scanner may not provide better specificity in readings for the low to mid-acuity patients that present at that hospital. In other words, the hospital would be unlikely to recover its investment because the additional technical capability is not warranted by the level of care offered. However, at a tertiary or quaternary level facility that offers subspecialty cardiac trauma, or neurosurgical care, it may make sense to invest in the highest possible level of technology. As a rule of thumb, technology should be thought of as a tool to leverage existing work processes rather than as an end in itself. Furthermore, many organizations overlook the clinical documentation systems that are needed to translate the outcomes of very high-tech laboratory, imaging, and surgical equipment into the organization's ongoing records systems.

There will always be tension between human resource and technology costs within health care organizations. The public often requests that hospitals make the high-tech investment in better, faster, and less invasive systems of care, holding onto the perception that the newest technology should be easily accessible at minimal cost—and those perceptions make sense based on the messages received from the media. In addition, because they have little to no idea of the investment or cost per use, the public has no price sensitivity for technology. Consumers of health care simply know that they want "the best."

Our task as leaders is to focus on the investments that will help us provide care that follows the Institute of Medicine (IOM) STEEP model—Safe, Timely, Efficient, Effective, and Patient centered. If it comes down to a choice between a bed-side information system that allows for real-time monitoring of laboratory results, pharmacy orders, physician orders, and test results, and a super-efficient linear accelerator that provides superior delivery of radiation oncology for only a handful of patients, the likelihood is that the clinical data system will be the better investment over time. Key to its success, though, is consistent use of the system to maximize data capture, enhance clinical performance, and decrease variations in care.

OTHER CONSIDERATIONS: USE OF TECHNOLOGY IN RECRUITING, STAFFING, AND SCHEDULING

Nurses initially encounter an organization's technology during the job search process. Their introduction to an organization may be through its Web site. Web sites and home pages may contain online application processes, automated skill assessments; general organizational information, as well as recent news about the facility. The Web site provides the prospective employee with a glimpse into the organization's approach to technology. These systems can vary greatly, from the simplest (a basic page listing job openings and a contact phone number) to the most advanced (virtual tours of the organization, online uploading of resumes, "job carts" of positions for which the candidate has applied, and recruitment videos featuring staff).

During the employee interview process, savvy job candidates may inquire about how technology is used for patient care and how it influences nurses' everyday work, including patient outcomes. Many job seekers (especially younger nurses who are more technologically astute) may use technology as a differentiator in their choice of employers. These more technologically astute individuals have been exposed to many types of technology in their academic and everyday life. They may see a hospital's technology as a proxy for its innovation and modernity. The opposite is also true: The less technologically astute job seeker who may not have had the same exposure to technology may see an organization's information systems as off-putting or intimidating. It is important that organizations understand the various perspectives job seekers may bring to technology in the workplace and be able to respond according to individual needs.

Another way in which staff immediately engage in the use of technology upon employment is through staffing and scheduling systems. These systems vary from stand alone systems that handle only staffing and scheduling, to those that are interconnected to payroll, time and attendance, productivity reporting, and resource management. Staffing schedules are developed based on a designated human resource budget that, in turn, is based on census and acuity requirements. The data used to identify these staffing needs are often retrieved from separate and disparate systems. For example, census is often based on the midnight patient count and therefore does not reflect the patient population during the peak time of the day. Therefore, staffing by shift, by acuity, by activity (how many admissions/discharges and transfers are expected during the shift), and census has greater accuracy in determining staff and patient care needs. Acuity systems that identify staffing needs have been based primarily on the use of manual assessment tools and applied periodically to ensure the validity of the process and tool. The technology surrounding staffing and scheduling frequently does not have an associated acuity feature built into the tool. Staffing and scheduling technology is only as good as the accessibility to staff. In the event the organization is experiencing a shortage of nurses or support personnel, it can be challenging to evaluate whether the employee with the right level of expertise is placed in the right setting at the right time, all the time.

Administratively, technology serves as the engine for the "bigger picture." It is important that systems have the capability to drill down to individual, unit, and organization-wide information. It is through technology that staff, leadership, administrators, and governing boards can plan, assess, evaluate, and operationally enhance the important work of the health care organization.

> "True transformation in health care will require a combination of strong leadership, process reengineering, and technology all complemented by a culture that is ready to embrace change. Technology can dramatically improve patient safety and quality while making caregiver workflow easier and more efficient."
>
> —Mary Beth Navarra-Sirio, RN, MBA;
> Vice President, Patient Safety and Quality,
> McKesson Corporation, Pittsburgh, Pennsylvania

CASE STUDY

A facility's policy and procedure manual states that "when a mother reaches 38 weeks' gestation, the physician-owned clinic will provide hard copy portions of the mother's prenatal record and send it in the interoffice mail to the labor and delivery nurses' station." This hard copy information is filed on the labor and delivery unit and used when the mother arrives for delivery. However, in the event the mother arrives prior to 38 weeks' gestation, little if any information is available to the labor and delivery staff or the on-call/attending physician.

The labor and delivery department recognized that an increasing number of mothers were entering for delivery during hours when the ambulatory clinic was not open. As a result, the staff and the on-call obstetrician did not have access to the patients' prenatal records, which are necessary in order to deliver optimal labor and delivery care. The unit nursing leadership convened a meeting with the chief nursing officer (CNO), the chief information officer (CIO), and the medical staff chairman of the OB/GYN department. The primary reason for the meeting was to discuss the concern surrounding patient safety due to lack of prenatal information from the physician-owned office. The entire team recognized that the presentation of mothers prior to 38 weeks' gestation to the labor and delivery were associated with an even higher risk. Through their discussion, the team agreed on the following three principles:

1. That the obstetric population was one of the highest volume admissions to the medical center.
2. That the obstetric population was subject to high liability.
3. That staff and physicians were "ready" for an automated approach to data-sharing for optimal patient care.

Working with the IT staff, they identified three vendors who could provide a potential solution. Each vendor was invited to showcase its system to staff, physicians, and leadership. A quantitative evaluation tool was developed (see Appendix) to assist in the determination of the vendor of choice based on various parameters.

After the systems were reviewed and the evaluations completed, the nursing staff determined that the "best of breed" vendor would be their top choice, as it had been used in the field the longest and had received high user ratings. Department leadership, however, chose a different vendor as their top choice because it allowed integration of the labor and delivery application with the postpartum mother–infant application. They concluded that this interoperability would provide for greater information flow after the mother transferred from labor and delivery to the postpartum unit. It would also provide for greater interoperability in the event the mother would require additional hospitalizations or outpatient services outside the admission for delivery. This particular vendor had only a few of these applications in the field and out of beta testing. The vendor offered the organization an excellent price for the application. With these accommodations, its product was both the lowest priced and the best integrated, although it was not the "best of breed" choice.

Based on budget constraints, the organization contracted with the integrated vendor. Several problems occurred upon installation. The vendor was very amenable to working out the solution and providing financial support. Based on the assessment questions below, what recommended changes or additions to the processes used by this department's staff and leadership, the CNO and CIO, would you suggest?

Assessment Questions

1. How do you know when a technology solution works well for an organization?
2. What technology solutions work well for you and your job responsibilities? Why?
3. How do you know when there is an opportunity to improve on current technology?
4. What technology solutions do not work well for you and why?
5. What workflows were used to study the technology needs of the department in this case study?
6. What were some of the issues associated with the various vendors?
7. When technology was recently installed in your facility, was workflow studied? Did workflow change after installation?
8. Did the technology improve the systems and processes that surrounded the care provided for the patient? Why or why not?
9. Who should participate in the technology assessment process?
10. Were you or a representative of your unit involved with the planning for technology needs as well as implementation of a recently acquired system or application?

Best Practice

- When technology solutions are being evaluated and implemented, it is important that nursing staff and leadership be present at the decision-making table.
- Ongoing evaluation is vital to ongoing technology success.
- Serve as a role model and mentor to existing staff and new staff.
- Develop and manage standards and behavior expectations for implementation and use.
- Develop job performance standards for the use of technology.
- Assist in developing metrics to evaluate the impact technology has on patient care process, patient outcomes, and provider satisfaction.

REFERENCES

1. Conn, Joseph. "Computers reduce odds of in-hospital deaths: Study", www. modernhealthcare.com. Modern Healthcares, Web article January 26, 2009.
2. Merian, Lucas."Obama's plans for health care IT: Too much money too soon?" Computer world, Feb 5, 2009.
3. Robinson, B. "States Accelerate Health IT Lawmaking." Government Health IT, December 10, 2008. Available at: http://govhealthit.com/Articles/2008/12/States-acceleratehealth-IT-lawmaking.aspx

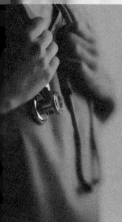

Chapter 6

ACADEMIA: THE VOICE OF PREPARATION

"If we are to foster a more seamless transition from academia to practice, we must engage in careful listening and sincere dialog. Each of us has something to offer, each has something to learn. In our effort to be right we may have forgotten that our mutual call is to lead through service."

—Sister Mariah Dietz, OSB, DNSc;
Director of Graduate Nursing,
University of Mary,
Bismarck, North Dakota

ACADEMIC PROGRAMS AVAILABLE FOR ASPIRING NURSE LEADERS

Degree Completion Programs for RNs (RN to BSN; RN to MSN)

Hundreds of bridge programs are offered for nurses with diplomas and associate of nursing (ADN) degrees who wish to complete a bachelor's or master's degree program in nursing. Many programs are offered online and in flexible formats designed for working nurses.

Master's Degree (MSN)

Master's degree programs prepare nurses for more independent roles such as nurse practitioner, clinical nurse specialist, nurse-midwife, nurse anesthetist, nurse administrator, or nurse psychotherapist. Master's-prepared nurses serve as expert clinicians, in faculty roles, and as specialists in geriatrics, community health, administration, nursing management, and other areas.

Doctoral Degree (PhD, EdD, DNS)

Doctoral programs prepare nurses to assume leadership roles within the profession, conduct research that influences nursing practice and health care, and teach at colleges and universities. Doctorally prepared nurses serve as health system executives, nursing school deans, researchers, practice experts, and senior policy analysts.

Postdoctoral Programs

Postdoctoral programs provide advanced research training for nurses who hold doctoral degrees. Currently, 24 research-focused universities across the country offer postdoctoral programs in nursing.

HISTORICAL OVERVIEW

In thinking about how we educate and prepare nurses and nurse leaders for current and future needs, it is important to remember where nursing started. The modern role of professional nursing is very different from its roots in the mid-nineteenth century. Florence Nightingale, perhaps the most famous nurse of all, began writing about nursing during her service in a British Army hospital in Turkey during the Crimean War. In 1859, she published the first textbook for nursing, entitled *Notes on Nursing: What it is and what it is not*. Nightingale was a pioneer in nursing, not only for her work to improve the practice of nursing, but also in her encouragement of nursing education. She organized the first nursing college, which is now part of King's College London. Prior to the founding of that school, nurses trained as apprentices, often as part of a religious order. Nightingale and her colleagues understood that nursing could be a viable career for lay persons and should be recognized for the science and theory that ground it. It was only through the efforts of Nightingale and other forward-thinking women that nursing became a licensed professional discipline.

Within 30 years of Nightingale's groundbreaking work, nurse training had grown exponentially. In 1873, the first nursing school in the United States opened at New York City's Bellevue Hospital. By 1879, there were 12 schools of nursing in the United States. In 1893, L. Dock with Isabel Hampton Robb and Mary Nutting founded the American Society of Superintendents of Training Schools for Nurses of the United States and Canada. This politically active organization became the National League for Nursing (NLN). Its mission statement states that the NLN "promotes excellence in nursing education to build a strong and diverse nursing workforce."[1]

In 1896, fewer than 20 nurses attended the first convention of the Nurses Associated Alumnae of the United States and Canada, which became, in 1911, the American Nurses Association.[2] Soon thereafter, Ms. Sophia Palmer, superintendent of the Rochester City Hospital School of Nursing and first editor of the *American Journal of Nursing* proposed state registration for training schools, in order to control the quality of nursing education.[3] By 1902, Miss Palmer and the New York State Nurses Association had advocated to have "Registered

Nurse" as the credential given to nurses who had graduated from state-licensed schools of nursing.[4]

In 1901, the U.S. Army Nurse Corps was founded, and in 1918, the Army School of Nursing was authorized by the secretary of war as an alternative to using nurses' aides in army hospitals. Nursing education programs immediately opened at several army hospitals.

Although nursing had always been open to men (in fact, Bellevue founded the first nursing school especially for men in 1888), the industry has traditionally been a women's field. During World War II, many women entered the workforce to fill the jobs of men who were deployed to the military. Once the war ended, women were once again relegated to traditional "service-oriented" roles, such as teaching and nursing.

EVOLUTION OF NURSING EDUCATION PROGRAMS

At the same time that the U.S. Army was developing its nursing education programs, the Rockefeller Foundation sought means to better train nurses for public health. The Foundation convened a committee that concluded (among other things):

> That . . . the average hospital training school is not organized on such a basis as to conform to the standards accepted in other educational fields; that the instruction in such schools is frequently casual and uncorrelated; that the educational needs and the health and strength of students are frequently sacrificed to practical hospital exigencies; that such shortcomings are primarily due to the lack of independent endowments for nursing education; that existing educational facilities are on the whole, in a majority of schools, inadequate for the preparation of the high grade of nurses required for the care of serious illness, and for service in the fields of public health nursing and nursing education.[4]

Thus, in 1923, Yale University started the first college-based nursing education program. Unlike hospital-based schools of nursing, the Yale program required its students to meet the academic standards of the university and to graduate with a baccalaureate degree. By the 1950s, Columbia University had instituted the first master's degree in a nursing clinical specialty.[5]

Despite these academic developments, until the 1970s most nurse trainings occurred in diploma programs associated with hospitals. Diploma programs were 3 years in length and focused on a great deal of time in the clinical setting. These programs trained nurses with the intention of keeping them as employees of the respective hospitals. Since the 1970s, many hospitals have transitioned their training programs to local universities and community colleges as a way of containing costs. Registered nurses are now educated and prepared through hundreds of associated degree baccalaureate degree and diploma programs throughout the nation.

As college-based programs became the norm, programs in nursing administration took a back seat to clinical specialty programs, including those for nurse practitioners. Thus, while many nurses developed specialized graduate degrees in midwifery or geriatric nursing, the management of nursing practice was not a part of the curriculum.

Today, many different levels and options for education exist, including traditional 4-year baccalaureate programs, bridge programs that enable associate and diploma degree RNs to obtain a BSN, accelerated programs at both the bachelor's and master's levels for those who already have degrees from other disciplines, traditional and specialized master's programs, dual master's programs (with business administration or health care administration), and doctoral programs. In addition, there are many different venue options, including on-campus learning, online programs, and programs that are offered on site at hospitals through colleges. Many nursing professional societies offer certification programs as well. In fact, the abundance of nursing education options has created confusion about the educational tracks that nurses should take. Both Johnson & Johnson and the Robert Wood Johnson Foundation have pledged support to create public access information resources to help prospective students navigate through the choices.

WHAT EDUCATION DOES AN ASPIRING NURSE LEADER NEED?

Many clinical areas provide only minimal leadership education. What little training does occur focuses on regulatory standards requiring a significant amount of highly technical information. However, when key national nurse leaders were interviewed, the majority of the leaders noted that they had enjoyed leadership opportunities at an early age. When they graduated from nursing school, they became recognized for their clinical competency. This automatically transferred a perception that, as highly skilled nurses, they would make excellent leaders.

The majority of the nursing leaders interviewed prior to writing this book had little, if any, formal education when they accepted their first nursing leadership opportunity. They learned on the job. In fact, it was not uncommon for a staff nurse to come to work on a particular shift and find himself or herself assigned the position of charge nurse for the unit due to a vacancy on that shift. Soon thereafter, the individual would be "tapped" by the leadership to consider a unit management position. Each of the leaders interviewed chose to pursue formal postgraduate education only after fulfilling a leadership role in these first-line supervisory positions for several years.[6]

New leaders need dedicated time to learn the various tools of leadership, and to establish those tools within their practice. No hospital would hire a surgeon without ensuring adequate training of the surgeon or providing a properly equipped operating room and tools for conducting surgery. Likewise, hospitals need to invest in the training and tools for nurse leaders to do their jobs.

In order to uphold a culture of professional practice, new nurse leaders need access to and support for education, development, and investment in leadership competencies. The programs that provide nursing leadership education (regardless of their format) are responsible for providing students with the

necessary knowledge and skills for the various roles they perform within the health care system.

NURSING PROFESSIONAL SOCIETIES RAISING THE BAR FOR NURSING LEADERSHIP

Over the past 20 years, numerous organizations have paved the
way for nursing leadership to blossom and mature. As they
uphold the role nurses play in health care, these organizations
also help to underscore the managerial- and executive-level
expertise needed to lead exemplary nursing organizations. The
Guiding Principles of the American Organization of Nursing
Executives (AONE) provide a framework for nursing leadership.
The American Association of Critical Care Nurses has written
extensively about healthy work environments. Most recently, the
NLN has issued position statements on processes for clinical
education.

Perhaps the most far-reaching of these efforts, however, is the
Magnet Recognition Program® of the American Nurses
Credentialing Center (ANCC). The hallmark of this program is
its identification of five model components that are structured to
focus health care organizations on achieving superior performance as evidenced by outcomes. These model components typify
the highest performing nursing organizations. The majority of
the standards for Magnet designation have to do with nursing
leadership, professionalism, and training. The Magnet standards
utilize empirical domains of evidence, which are further
described through the Magnet model components. The five components are:

1. Transformational leadership.

2. Structural empowerment.

3. Exemplary professional practice.

4. New knowledge, innovations, and improvements.

5. Empirical quality outcomes.

Within each of these components are sources of evidence that describe and provide the evidence of meeting these standards. Facilities that achieve Magnet designation have higher rates of baccalaureate- and master's-prepared nurses, as well as higher rates of professional society participation. Today there are 321 Magnet-designated facilities in 43 states.[8] Accreditation speaks to an enormous organizational commitment to quality patient care and nursing excellence.

CONTINUING THE EVOLUTION OF NURSING EDUCATION AND LEADERSHIP DEVELOPMENT

What the Rockefeller Foundation commission concluded nearly a century ago is still true today. The public need for highly trained nurses (and nurse leaders) requires that training programs provide consistent high-quality, comprehensive academic preparation. It is incumbent on accrediting bodies to recognize the knowledge, skills, and competencies necessary to provide and manage care in a complex health care system. An additional factor to consider is that most tuition for nurse leaders is paid for by hospitals employing those nurses. Therefore, hospitals want to ensure the value of their educational investments.

It behooves both the schools of nursing and health care organizations to respond and collaborate on ways to minimize duplication and remove "silos" within curricula. Savvy nursing school deans recognize that hospitals serve a function beyond simply providing a clinical rotation site for students. Hospitals are both the supplier of students and the "purchaser" of the colleges' finished product: graduate nurses. Therefore, colleges are working harder to ensure that the programs they offer better meet the needs of hospitals, as well as students.

Collaboration is important for faculty development as well. One of the leading constraints to expanding nursing education programs is the shortage of faculty. Simply put, individuals with

the qualifications to be nursing faculty can make more as practitioners than they can as teachers. To address this issue, colleges and hospitals can work together to create employment
scenarios that reward employees for joint practice as both
advanced practitioners and faculty.

Likewise, one of the best ways in which schools of nursing
can collaborate with hospitals is by emphasizing collaborative
practice—both within the academic setting and within the
clinical setting. Several collaborative care models exist; these
ought to be central to all clinical education tracks. Rather than
providing education in "silos," academia needs to become
proactive and develop curriculum and collaborative care models that teach health care teams to reduce variability, improve
communication, and strive for positive patient outcomes.

Vanderbilt University Professor Peter Buerhaus is one of the
nation's champions for interdisciplinary workforce development. In a 2009 webinar, Buerhaus suggested that health care
reimbursement and academic intuitions should both be tied to
whether the organizations teach collaborative practice.[9]
Through his work at Vanderbilt, Buerhaus seeks to bring the
study of medicine, social work, physical therapy, occupational
therapy, respiratory care and nursing into multidisciplinary
courses that allow budding practitioners to work together. In
this way, students participate in collaborative teams that mirror
how patient care planning occurs and is best facilitated.
Buerhaus and his colleagues ask, "If this is not a part of the education and training, how can the individual discipline be successful in the work environment?"

Another way in which nursing schools can collaborate with
hospitals is to increase the teaching focus on regulatory and
reimbursement issues. Many of the pay-for-performance indicators being touted by the Centers for Medicare and Medicaid
Services are nursing-centric. Therefore, graduate nurses will
have immediate responsibility and accountability to practice
according to the payer and regulatory requirements.

Nursing schools can also work with hospitals to evaluate
and respond to the trends within the nursing workforce. For

instance, in response to the increasing number of nurses over 50, nursing leadership programs may want to spend time educating and preparing students about the ergonomic and communication needs of older employees. Classroom discussions on technology may incorporate a review of best practices in technology adoption for older users. Similarly, with more foreign-born nurses, leadership programs may want to pay attention to the ways in which cultural differences may influence team dynamics, patient communication, and ethical decision making.

As reinforcement of this collaboration, the Joint Commission on Accreditation of Healthcare Organizations requires that faculty from schools of nursing and leaders from clinical rotation sites meet regularly. Working together, the schools and clinical sites are expected to seek common ways to enhance the student experience, discuss current issues at the forefront, review relevant policy changes, and ensure that the transition from student nurse to registered nurse meets or exceeds the expectations of both the new hire and the organization. This relationship and ongoing communication can yield great results professionally and academically.

SPECIAL CONSIDERATION FOR NURSING LEADERSHIP CURRICULA

One of the key tenets of this book is that nurse leaders need the proper business and managerial skills to meet organizational goals. Therefore, the following are key skills and areas of concentration within nursing leadership training programs:

1. *Business acumen.* Nurse leaders must be able to make good managerial and finance decisions, and to participate in multidisciplinary teams to drive business objectives. Specific to the responsibilities of the nurse leader is the fact that a medical floor, for example, can be synonymous with a multimillion dollar business. Clinical as well as business competencies provide for successful operations.

2. *Value-based measurement and reporting.* Nurse leaders need to be able to articulate the value of the nursing care provided by their organization (whether within a unit, division, service line, or the entire hospital). Nurse leaders must understand how to measure, evaluate, and act on nurse-sensitive indicators, knowing full well *how* nursing interventions (or lack there of) have a direct impact on these indicators. They must be adept in quality improvement and process monitoring. They should hone both quantitative and qualitative skills to review and report on performance.

3. *Strong assessment, data use, and communication skills.* Leaders make decisions by studying facts, formulating plans of action, and driving the execution of the plan. Therefore, nurse leaders must be able to quickly identify and understand a problem, as well as to make decisions in a fair, thoughtful, and decisive way. How nurse leaders communicate is often the most important factor in their leadership success: They must learn the importance and value of being trustworthy, honest, and clear in their communications, and must become proficient in motivating staff to gain commitment.

4. *Competency assessment and planning.* Nurse leaders must constantly evaluate the competencies of their staff and make plans to ensure individual and team performance that results in high-quality, efficient, low-cost care. When staff need competency development, nurse leaders must be able to recognize the need and provide ongoing opportunities for skill development and mastery. Leaders must also evaluate the learning needs of new staff and ensure competency development in order to minimize frustration that might lead to staff turnover.

5. *Cultural awareness and relationship management.* Nurse leaders are some of the most important people helping to shape the culture and relationships within hospital work areas. With proper training, nurse leaders can quickly identify opportunities to build team rapport and to reinforce a cohesive, healthy work culture. In a strong positive culture, staff may say, "When I arrive at work and find that Kendra and I are assigned to the

same team and provided patient assignments, I know my day will be a great day. We work together as a team, we communicate, and the patients recognize our teamwork." Whereas, in a culture that may not be as optimally healthy, staff may say, "When I come to work and see that I have been assigned to work with Kristen, I brace myself for a day that involves carrying the majority of the workload and performing most of the care to our assigned patients. I become resentful, and at the end of the day, I leave hoping I have provided the necessary care to my patients." The leadership's contribution and recognition to growing and sustaining a healthy work culture is key to quality patient care and professional engagement.

A WORD ON NURSING LEADERSHIP THEORY

Most nursing schools include some type of leadership and management course or lessons in the curriculum. These courses may present a single theory of nursing leadership or review a variety of theories. Once aware of the existing theories, a nurse can subscribe to whichever best fits her or his personality. A nurse leader should choose the leadership theory that best reflects his or her ideals and can be used effectively. No one rates the theories; each one has pros and cons. Once ascribed to, however, the theory should be reinforced. Followup is often inconsistent, despite senior leaders saying their priority is creating active leaders for the future of health care. Senior leaders can help their younger colleagues by inviting discussions of leadership theory, as well as constant review and updating of the theory's application in practice.

This chapter's focus is on the history of nursing education and the evolving role that academia and schools of nursing have on nurse training and leadership development. We know that having an adequate and competent workforce is vital to positive patient outcomes. Ensuring access to thorough, comprehensive training is the key to preparing nurse leaders.

"Patients are getting the right care overall; however, I am not certain they are getting the right care in the right order. Staff require the skill set necessary to address the needs of today. Education is complex and a great deal is expected of new graduates. Existing staff have grown up with the technology we currently utilize. We need internships or residencies to help with the new graduate transition to the current environment. Academia needs to emphasize the educational needs of their students given the complex environment. The concept of joint appointments with defined criteria and expectation to keep faculty competent in the field is vital."

–Terry Watne, MS, RN; Administrative Director, Altru Health System, Grand Forks, North Dakota

CASE STUDY

Susan was a bright-eyed graduate nurse who was hired to work on a 10-bed oncology unit. She was excited to land a job at her first-choice hospital, and on the unit where she desired to work. Susan's interview was brief, lasting only about 15 minutes. At the time, there were four registered nurse openings on the unit. Susan asked only a few questions because she was so excited to have the chance to apply for a position doing what she loved. Susan was passionate about oncology, because both her grandmother and mother had died from breast cancer in their mid-Forties.

Susan arrived at the hospital for her first day of work and was instructed to go to the auditorium for hospital orientation. Twenty-two employees attended this orientation, and Susan was one of three graduate/registered nurses in the orientation group. The rest of the employees were nurse assistants, respiratory care technicians, a social worker, a new manager, and two physical therapists.

Susan had a brief opportunity to meet the other nursing colleagues; however, they were hired for and assigned to different nursing units and shifts so she rarely saw them again after that first day. On day 2, Susan was met on the oncology unit by the unit nursing educator. The educator provided "just-in-time" orientation, which meant that she gave Susan her locker code, advised her on the location of the bathroom, and provided the codes to access the medication room, the automated medication administration device, and the computerized charting system. The unit educator provided Susan with an overview of the unit-based policies and procedures document describing the operational scope of the oncology unit.

Gloria, a seasoned registered nurse who had worked on the oncology unit for the past 9 years, was then assigned to Susan as her buddy for the next 2 days. Gloria provided Susan with the best "on-the-job" orientation possible. Susan had a checklist, but Gloria commented, "Oh, I'm aware of that tool, but just follow me, you'll learn to do your own thing in time."

Susan observed numerous workarounds occurring over the course of her next 2 days. She adapted to the culture of the unit and before long "became one of them" so that she would "fit in with the group" and not have to deal with colleagues talking behind her back. She wanted to be accepted as part of the staff on the unit.

Susan also observed that the physicians who practiced on this nursing unit were very influential and demanded that care be provided per their direction only. Informally, Susan was told by her colleagues that should not disturb Drs. Miller or Jonah in the middle of the night unless she wanted to be "hung out to dry" the next day when they made rounds. Susan was told to wait until the morning to contact these two physicians for care orders for their patients.

Assessment Questions

1. What gaps can you identify in the processes to which Susan was exposed?
2. What principles would you embrace as a leader for that unit?
3. Was Susan's experience like your own experience as a new employee? Why or why not?
4. What might the unit leaders do to ensure that Susan has a better experience going forward?
5. What might Susan's academic program have done to prepare her for her interview and new employee experiences?

Best Practice

- Academic programs in nursing have evolved significantly over the past century, with most changes occurring in the past 40 years.
- Nursing professional societies are advancing the professionalism and centrality of nursing leadership.
- Collaboration is a key element in nursing education.
- Nursing leadership education must focus on competency assessment, communication, business acumen, and relationship management.
- Nursing schools and hospitals have the opportunity to collaborate on education programs and faculty development.

REFERENCES

1. National League for Nursing Web site. Available at: http://www.nln.org

2. American Nurses Association Web site. Available at: http://www.ana.org

3. "History of The Rochester City Hospital Training School for Nurses." Available at: http://www.viahealth.org/body_rochester.cfm?id=711

4. Varney, H. Yale School of Nursing: A Brief History, p. 5. Available at: http://www.med.yale.edu/library/nursing/historical/shorthist/NursingHistory.pdf

5. "Columbia University: The School of Nursing Description and History." Available at: http://www.nursing.columbia.edu/about-school/history.html

6. Campbell, C. (2000). Personal Communication. June 2008.

7. Ross, A. Wenzel, F. J., Mitlyng, J. W. (2001). Leadership for the Future, Health Administration Press, AUPHA Press, Chicago.

8. American Nurses Credentialing Center Web site. Available at: http://www.nursecredentialing.org/Magnet/FindaMagnetFacility.aspx

9. "State of the State with Dr. Peter Buerhaus: The Latest Projections of Nursing's Future." webinar, presented January 29, 2009. Available at: http://www.concerro.com/webcasts/webcast_20081218.htm

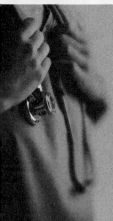

Chapter 7

PLANNING FOR LEADERSHIP AND SUPPORTING NEW LEADERS

"We are gardeners; we have the responsibility to tend to our organizations, facilitating their growth and development, for our future generations. We have the responsibility to develop care models, promote diversity, achieve good patient outcomes, ensure affordable and fiscally sound health care, and develop staff. We will be judged on how well we prepare our health care systems for those who follow in our footsteps."

—Deborah Zimmermann, MS, RN, NEA-BC; Rochester, New York; Board of Directors, Magnet Commission, Silver Spring, Maryland

THE FUTURE NURSE LEADER

The preceding chapters provide a high-level framework for students, faculty, aspiring nurse leaders, and current nurse leaders to understand the issues facing health care today and the impact that leadership has on the role of the nurse of the future. The knowledge and skill sets acknowledged in this book cover a wide variety of subjects. My intent was to provide a pathway for exploring and further enhancing nursing leadership and the vital role that nursing plays in the future of health care in the United States.

At the beginning of the book, I described leadership and the roles of leaders within hospitals. In this chapter, I focus on the ways in which organizations can identify and support new leaders in their midst.

PLANNING FOR LEADERSHIP

Within most hospitals, human resources account for well over 50% of the total budget. Nursing is usually the largest human resource budget line, representing up to two thirds of the entire personnel budget. Nursing budgets and staffing patterns can flex up or down, depending on census and acuity, but the overall nursing budget is a "sunk cost" that hospitals incur regardless of the number or types of patients that come through the door. Although human capital is the most expensive aspect of the organization, it is also the most important. Health care is a knowledge- and service-based commodity in which various clinical expert disciplines contribute to the multidisciplinary care of the patient.

Key aspects of human resources are access, recruitment, retention, allocation, competence and management. The development of a human resource plan is integral to the success of any organization, and especially important to leadership identification, training, and support.

We have already identified that the face of nursing is different than it was 30 years ago; today's nurses are older and more of them hail from different nations and cultures. In order to ensure that adequate and competent staffs are assigned to care for patients, it is imperative that health care organizations use a nursing resource management plan. These plans include all aspects of an organization's human resource plan, including the additional components or goals (or both) that are specific to nursing.

Nursing resource management plans should be a direct reflection of the personnel needs that contribute to patient care outcomes. Most often we think of personnel needs as they relate to direct patient care. However, a well-developed nursing resource management plan will also review and incorporate nursing-specific domains such as unit and department management; quality improvement, patient safety, and research; informatics and data base management; education and clinical resource support; and budget and fiscal management.

UNDERSTANDING THE DATA THAT DRIVE NURSING RESOURCE MANAGEMENT PLANS

Chief nursing officers and other leaders find it best to use a data-driven, proven tool for ongoing needs assessment and plan development.

The basic building block for the nursing resource management plan is average census. Keep in mind that patient census varies throughout the day. Fiscal budgets report midnight census whereas the greatest activity on a patient care unit occurs between 9 a.m. and 7 p.m. For example, a unit might commonly have a midnight census of 22 one day and the next day at midnight, 25. Although it appears that only 2 patients were admitted during that period, the real story of patient flow is quite different. It would not be uncommon to see 10 patients discharged and 12 new patients admitted!

As lengths of stay continue to shorten, the way in which nurses provide care for patients is also changing. Nursing care is now a much more intense process than it was in the past, with more people interacting with the patient over shorter periods of time. Further, because occupancy is rising as lengths of stay decrease, nurses see more patients per shift than they did in the past. Therefore, the nursing resource management plan must also take into account the relative severity of illness or acuity of the patients within each unit. In my experience, the mode census, along with the frequency of the daily patient turnover, yields the best outcome for concurrent as well as staffing budgeting projected needs.

A patient in an ambulatory setting has far different needs that one in the intensive care unit or the labor and delivery unit. Likewise, the leadership skills and needs will be different on each of these units. Each specialty of nursing (emergency, surgical, obstetrics, etc.) has a professional organization that has studied both the type of staffing and types of leadership that are most effective in their respective settings. Nursing resource management plans should incorporate the recommendations of the respective societies in order to provide evidence-based practice in staffing and leadership development.

As exemplar resources, professional organizations provide nurses with many of the tools necessary to grow personally and professionally. They also provide tool kits, best practices, position statements, and access to almost anything an individual needs. These professional organizations also provide opportunities for dialogue as it relates to our future as nurses. What might the role of the nurse of the future look like? Utilize these excellent resources and committed professionals.

In summary then, the nursing resource management plan should incorporate the average daily census, mode census, daily patient turnover, and professional society recommendations specific to each nursing specialty. The plan should have two key sections. The first comprises the short-term elements that speak to the staffing needs and contingency resources that will be deployed in the event of an emergency. The second describes the nursing leadership needs of the respective units and departments, including plans to foster individual development as leaders.

ASSESSING CULTURES WITHIN THE NURSING UNITS FOR THE ASPIRING NURSE LEADER

What steps should a nursing department take when individuals demonstrate qualities that might make them good leaders? Perhaps the most important and valuable thing that can happen is to provide an assessment of the knowledge and skills of the individual. Not every individual has leadership acumen in all areas. Some might show more talent in clinical leadership, while other might have a better basis for organizational management. To create the most opportunities for success, it benefits both the individual and the organization to carefully assess and discern the individual's skills and interests and to train the individual accordingly. In addition, both an assigned mentor and regular scheduled meetings with the novice leader's supervisor assist in assessing the individual's progression.

It may be in the best interest of the organization to enlist outside assistance in the development of the novice leader. Many national programs provide leadership growth opportunities. Outside leadership education can be most rewarding and influential in personal and professional growth. One of my faculty colleagues shared that individuals attending such programs, value the programs for both the content and the camaraderie they provide. Within these settings, novice leaders will find similar levels of competency and the safety to explore the material in an open, discursive way. After the program is over, participants also benefit from a new network of colleagues with whom to further enhance leadership growth.

Keep in mind that, as leaders develop and refine their skill sets, organizations need to grow with them. Although formal individual training is a key building block to success, another important element is the work environment. Simply stated, empowering environments foster leadership, and environments that diminish independence and creativity will stifle the individual professional's growth. The one variable that will influence the environment most is the nurse leader; through her or his example, other nurses glean a sense of vision, purpose, value, and overall professionalism. Nurse leaders drive nursing satisfaction, which drives culture, which drives patient outcomes and satisfaction. The culture that nurse leaders create, as well as support, is palpable to everyone who enters the unit.

As you walk through the doors of any institution, you immediately gain a sense as to how the organization operates. When the physical environment is clean, you have a sense of safety and security. When bulletin boards describe quality improvement efforts, personal successes of the staff, and community health activities, you have a sense that employees take pride in their workplace and their roles. When you are greeted with a smile or asked whether you need directions to get to your destination, you sense that the employees care about you as a person. These are just a few clues to an organization's culture.

Nurses can just as easily assess the culture of their units, although the questions may be more technical. Questions they may ask include: What is the unit nursing turnover rate? What indicators of quality and performance does this particular unit exhibit? What do the staff of the unit like best about their work? Over the past 2 years, what goals have they accomplished and what role do those goals play within the division of nursing? As nurses evaluate the professional contribution and the impact they have on quality patient care, they will also decide how involved they want to be as leaders within the unit, and as supporters of leadership initiatives.

High-performing units and departments often approach development in tandem: they look at both the skills of their individuals and the culture of the overall work setting. This approach makes good sense on a number of levels—if the individual tries to apply new skills to an organization that is not culturally open to new thinking, that individual will fail. Likewise, if the culture seems to want innovation, it will stall if the leader does not have the skills to foster the new activities.

Often a particular unit serves as the "pilot unit" or incubator for new processes, approaches, and policies. The adaptability of that particular department speaks to its culture and leadership, both of which introduce and encourage change as a means to improve and streamline the complex systems in health care.

USING THE NURSING RESOURCE MANAGEMENT PLAN TO FOSTER NOVICE NURSES AND LEADERS

As described earlier, a hospital may embrace many different facets of leadership development that fall along a continuum from committee participation to formal academic training. The National Advisory Council on Nurse Education and Practice[1] calls for at least two thirds of the nurse workforce to hold baccalaureate or higher degrees in nursing by 2010. Currently, only 47.2% of nurses hold degrees at the baccalaureate level and above.[2]

Whether returning to school for their BSN or newly graduated from a BSN program, most nurses begin their careers in the acute care setting. Every novice nurse and novice leader wants to use his or her skills to add value within the clinical setting. However, as many seasoned nurse leaders will agree, "you only know what you know." In other words, the classroom teaches many things, but there are many intrinsic elements of nursing and leadership that are learned only with experience. The acute care setting is the most complex of all practice settings and requires numerous competencies beyond formal education. Again, nurse leaders within the hospital can act as mentors and guides for these staff nurses as they expand their knowledge of professional nursing practice.

For practicing nurses who return to school to obtain a BSN, pursuing that degree represents a leadership journey in itself. Nurses who return to school recognize that they are expanding their knowledge base to further themselves and their role in patient care. Many times, the work that nurses do in the classroom leads to a higher level of inquiry and engagement in their clinical settings. Recognizing and supporting that engagement is key to fostering the individual's role as a leader.

Evidence and published research find that the baccalaureate-prepared nurse has a significant impact on patient care. Research conducted by Linda Aiken, PhD, of the University of Pennsylvania found that the odds of dying are reduced from 44% to 19% when staff registered nurses are prepared at the BSN level. The research also indicated that the odds of dying were reduced by 16% when 60% of staff held BSNs versus 20%.[3] Aiken and colleagues reported their findings in the *Journal of the American Medical Association*. They noted that each 10% increase in the proportion of nurses with BSNs was associated with a 5% decline in the mortality following common surgical procedures. Also noted was the fact that each 10% increase in BSNs was associated with a 5% decline in failure to rescue.[3] Their evidence suggests that a smaller, more highly educated nurse workforce could achieve outcomes comparable with a larger, less well-educated workforce.

Because of the significant expense associated with the extensive orientation and education of new staff, nursing resource management plans must also assess how new nurses (and new nurse leaders) will be supported and retained during the earliest part of their career.

As an aside, accessing local, state, and national leadership organizations can provide a wealth of knowledge, skills, networking, and growth opportunities. The following is not an exhaustive list; however, it includes organizations whose commitment to both leadership and clinical competencies I have witnessed firsthand.

- American Organization of Nurse Executives: http://www.aone.org.
- American College of Healthcare Executives: http://www.ache.org.
- Emergency Nurses Association: http://www.ena.org
- American Association of Critical Care Nurses: http://www.aacn.org.
- American Nurses Association: http://www.ana.org
- National Association for Healthcare Quality: http://www.nahq.org.

- American Nurses Credentialing Center: http://www.nursecredentialing.org
- American Organization of Perioperative Nurses: http://www.aorn.org
- Agency for Healthcare Research and Quality: http://www.ahrq.gov
- Leap Frog Group: http://www.leapfroggroup.org
- Institute for Healthcare Improvement: http://www.ihi.org

COMMUNICATION AND NURSING LEADERSHIP: THE FOUNDATION FOR INTEGRITY AND TRUST

It has been said that high-quality health care is about delivering the right care to the right patient in the right way at the right time. In many ways, the same axiom can be applied to nursing leadership. Instead of patient care, however, the context involves communication: high-quality leadership is about conveying the right words to the right person in the right way at the right time.

Not everyone is born with an innate sense of how to communicate well. We all have moments when we struggle to communicate complex ideas, difficult messages, or concise statements. The complicated, fragmented world of nursing only adds to this difficulty. Many chief nursing officers can relay funny, touching, and sometimes painful stories of their early nursing careers and the lessons they learned about communicating with patients, families, staff, and physicians. They will each say that it took time, and they will probably point to a mentor whom they emulated, or who was kind enough to coach them on proper communication technique.

When nurses move into leadership, we assume they will know how to communicate in this new role. Just as nurses learn how to communicate as patient care professionals, nurse leaders need to learn how to communicate their new role with confidence, decisiveness, and humility. Both the words they use and the manner in which they communicate will have a significant bearing on their success in the role.

FOUR KEY COMMUNICATION CAPABILITIES

There are four areas in particular where new nurse leaders often need to learn effective communication techniques. First and foremost, nurse leaders must be aware of and responsive to, the weight and influence of what they communicate as leaders. I always encourage new nurse leaders to remember that their role as a leader does not make them better or more important than any other member of the team. Rather, as a leader, they have a duty to remain humble, to gather and assess information objectively, and to incorporate the perspective of direct care nurses in every decision they make. It is not always easy to remain objective, especially when executive leaders make decisions with which an individual leader does not agree. It can also be challenging to lead those who once were peers and friends. The friendships do not need to end, but the role of nurse leader does require that at work, a boundary be drawn. Not everything should be shared with the staff, and not every staff concern should be taken to the executive level. Discretion, professionalism, and consistency are the hallmarks of good communication with other nurses.

The second piece of communication wisdom for new managers is the skill of "managing up." When a nurse leader manages up, she or he gives credit to the individuals who have been role models and teachers for that nurse leader. Managing up does two things: it shows the rest of the team that even leaders need to learn, and it lets aspiring nurse leaders know that they will be supported in their own career journeys. Managing up is a way of injecting humility and humanity into the leadership role. Developing this skill is especially important for new nurse leaders, who may be insecure in their new roles and likely to overemphasize their authority. Managing up also creates opportunities to celebrate other individuals or groups within the organization that are doing exemplary things. In recognizing those individuals, the leader sends the message that success is driven by the team, and that every person and group has the capacity to excel.

What happens if managing up is not used? Two things tend to occur. First, if leaders do not acknowledge the positive influence that others have made on them and on the organization, they risk being seen as callous, egotistical, or unapproachable. Second, without the celebration of others, the respective pieces of the organization may lose sight of the big picture and begin to think in "silos."

I encountered an interesting example of silos at a nurse's day celebration a few years ago. That year, we encouraged each of the nursing units to describe and celebrate its accomplishments for the year, as well as current and future goals. On the day of the celebration, each unit turned out in force. One of the units was quite small; it only had 25 staff members. Even so, they invited their physicians to the celebration, and to their great joy, two physicians attended the event. Later those physicians told the nurses how astounded they were by the profound and many ways in which nurses throughout the medical center were touching and healing patients and families. The physicians' interest and pride in their colleagues was very apparent, and it really highlighted the ways in which isolation within one area can develop false perceptions among the team.

The third communication skill is to relay information thoroughly and in a timely manner. Many times, these important elements of communication get lost simply because of the vast amounts of information that flow back and forth in hospitals. As a result, communication is consistently one of the lowest scoring items on staff satisfaction surveys. Yet, when given the feedback they need to communicate better, nurse leaders often respond, "But I talk to the nurses all the time!" Effective communication depends on what is said, when, and how.

As an example, consider the communication that occurs between nurses and patients. Despite all the technology available today, patients frequently are asked the same question multiple times by different members of the health care team.

At the same time, it is not uncommon for a nurse to go in and out of patient rooms up to 75 times during a 12-hour shift. The average communication between nurse and patient during one of those 75 trips is 30 seconds. Again, the issue is not with the number of interactions. Rather, the issue is with the brevity of the communications. In order to communicate well, staff nurses as well as nurse leaders must slow down, communicate in full sentences, make sure that the listener understands, and seek confirmation of what was said.

In fact, one of my colleagues recalled that when she was a new vice president, the mantra her CEO kept repeating to her was: "Slow down! When you talk and move so quickly, it creates anxiety in your team." Nurses understand that their leaders are busy, but nothing is more frustrating than getting only a piece of the information, or getting it late. Nurse leaders may find it useful to leave phone messages and send well-worded e-mails to reinforce things that are said in passing. A phone message sent to clarify an incomplete communication might include the following points:

> Mary, earlier today I asked you about the timing mechanisms on the IV pumps. You may have wondered why I was asking. Tony in biomedical engineering said that some of the staff in the perfusion center have had timing mechanism glitches, and I wonder what your experience has been? Could you let me know by Tuesday? We'll be discussing it at the equipment committee meeting on Wednesday, and if it's a widespread issue, we'll need to respond. Thanks for your help on this.

Likewise, the following e-mail example shows how a nurse leader might recognize an individual for work on a special project:

> John, I know we didn't get to your item on the clinical standards committee agenda today. It's clear that you'd done a lot of preparation for that meeting, and I don't want it to get lost between now and the next meeting. Let's sit down on Friday for 10 minutes to review two or three of the top recommendations. Perhaps there is something we can do informally prior to full committee review and approval. Thanks.

Whether communicating with unit staff, or communicating with senior executives, board members, community representatives, or policy makers, relaying information calmly, thoroughly, and in a timely manner is a vital skill for nurse leaders to cultivate.

The fourth and final element of nursing leadership communication pertains to physician interaction. In many organizations, the nursing staff and the medical staff have a difficult, if not actually contentious, relationship. The American Nurses Association's scope and standards of nursing practice are very clear about the role that nurses are to play in hospital care: physicians order and direct patient care, and nurses execute and manage it.

As we all know, however, keen nurses continuously assess the need for changes in the plan of care. In order to perform these highly complex functions, the nurse develops a trajectory of cognitive and intuitive skills, as outlined in Benner's novice-to-expert model. As a new graduate, the staff nurse cannot be expected to function at the same level as the nurse who has been in the same role for 1, 2, or even 10 years.

The same is true for nurse leaders. Nurse leaders assess the need for change within the hospital unit, department, nursing division, and hospital as a whole. Novice leaders need time to develop and hone these skills, and part of their skill development includes assessing nursing interactions with physicians. Early in their careers, nurse leaders may be intimidated by medical staff members and physician leadership. However, successful nurse leaders overcome that intimidation to work effectively with physicians in planning for and managing effective, high-quality patient care. It may help new nurse leaders to remember that physicians had to learn their role, too. In my experience, most physicians are data driven and logical, and they will respond to information if it is presented in a way that is concise, thorough, and accurate. Physicians also appreciate information that is contextualized. They tend to think in the short term, and they tend to be solution driven. Thus, for example, when discussing operating room block times with the chief of surgery, she or he is more likely to "hear" what is being said during a meeting specific to scheduling than as an aside in a meeting scheduled for other purposes.

In reviewing each of these four communication examples (maintaining humility/objectivity, managing up, providing deliberate/timely communications, and demonstrating empowered physician interaction), the key question to ask is, How would I feel if I was receiving this information? Often the best route is to pause and reflect on how information might be misinterpreted. From there, the nurse leader can shape the message to ensure understanding and engagement that will minimize misunderstandings.

Make a conscious effort to ask open-ended questions, that is, questions starting with the words "how" or "what": How do you see this situation? What are your thoughts? These types of questions seek input and convey to other people or groups that you are interested and value their opinions. They also tend to yield a wealth of information. By soliciting input, they send the message that you care, and this is a motivating influence for many people.

When you communicate with an individual who reports to you, formally or informally, make a conscious effort to obtain his or her opinion before you provide yours. Giving your opinion first automatically thrusts the other individual into a defensive position, particularly when she or he disagrees.

Hospitals can support the communication skills of new leaders in a number of ways. Some hospitals provide classes to enhance communication skills and the tools necessary to ensure consistency in communication approaches. These classes may include topics such as oral communication, written documentation, and presentation, phone etiquette, and even scripting of certain key conversations such as disciplinary reviews. Other organizations use nurse leader shadowing, mentoring, or peer group formats to provide opportunities to model communication styles. Yet others simply provide a set of communication standards and let the novice leaders incorporate those standards on their own. Regardless of the delivery method, hospitals should do what they can to recognize and support the development of communication skills in new nurse leaders.

> *"Encourage self-development with opportunities outside the nurses' comfort zone. Assist in role modeling and applying the global perspective versus an individual or unit-based perspective. Articulate in terms of 'connecting the dots' so that standards, actions, accountability, and outcome are components of the entire picture."*
>
> —Judith K. Walker, MS, RN, NEA-BC, PLNC;
> Past President, AONE Council of Nurse Managers.
> Firestone, Colorado

CASE STUDY

This case study can be used to mentor new nurse leaders. Ken was a 51-year-old healthy man who required orthopedic surgery that could not be performed in his home town. With preadmission documents in hand, Ken and his wife Mary flew to the city where the referring hospital was located, arriving the night before surgery. They stayed at a local hotel and the next morning arrived at the hospital at 6 a.m. They were greeted by a volunteer at the front desk, who provided directions to the OR waiting room where, within 5 minutes, an RN took Ken and Mary back to the private preoperative prep room. The RN explained to Ken and Mary what each could expect over the course of the next few hours. The nurse provided a number of cares to Ken and offered various relaxation amenities, such as aromatherapy and music therapy. A cotton ball scented with lavender was taped to the chest of Ken's gown, the lights in the prep room were dimmed and serene, and calming music played. When it was time for Ken to go into the OR, the nurse gave Mary a pager and told her that it would work anywhere on the hospital campus. The nurse also advised Mary that she would be paged within 5 minutes of the end of Ken's surgery, at which point the surgeon would meet her in the OR waiting room to discuss the results.

The surgery was successful, and the surgeon met with Mary to discuss Ken's case and his recovery. After a period of time in the postanesthesia care unit, Ken was brought to his official patient room where he would stay for the next 3 nights. He was assessed by the nurses on the unit, who provided information to Mary about his care plan and the elements of his recovery. The nurses also described a process improvement project on the unit, which could involve student nurses observing while care was provided to Ken during his stay. Throughout his stay on the unit, Ken and Mary played an integral role in the plan for care and discharge. Mary even made a point of documenting Ken's discharge plan on the white board in his room. It read:

Discharge Plan

1. Patient and wife must be at the airport no later than 0600 on Wednesday, January 10.
2. Discharge prescriptions that require filling—please provide to wife by Tuesday p.m.
3. Discharge teaching for medication administration (self-administered blood thinner, pain medication) and physical therapy—please complete by Tuesday p.m.

Although Mary's decisive plan elicited several chuckles over the course of the 3-day stay, every member of the health care team understood what was needed to make the discharge happen without a problem or a delay.

Assessment Questions

1. Describe the elements of communication that Ken and Mary experienced.
2. Many of the behaviors of the staff seemed to be part of their "normal operating procedure." How did the staff know how and what to communicate?
3. What might an experienced nurse leader want to point out to a new nurse leader to ensure that this level of communication occurs in all settings?
4. What specific elements of education, service, quality, and safety did you observe in the communications?
5. How could nursing leadership support the continued development of communication skills among the hospital staff?

Best Practice

- Recognize that each encounter requires a planned, systematic means of execution. This includes scheduling, arrival, throughput, communication, and patient/family experience.
- Including the patient and family in the plan of care is vital.
- Utilization of visual cues for the entire health care team, including patient and family, creates consistent expectations.
- Consider asking the patient and family what their expectations are of their visit or hospitalization.
- Discharge begins the minute the patient enters the door of the facility. Inquiry and education are vital facets of the discharge plan. "Ken, your hospitalization is expected to be 3 days. Is there anything I, as your nurse, and other members of the health care team need to know that may be a barrier to your discharge on Wednesday?"

REFERENCES

1. National Advisory Council on Nurse Education and Practice Web site. Available at: http://bhpr.hrsa.gov/nursing/nacnep.htm
2. American Association of Colleges of Nursing fact sheet, September 2008. Available at: http://www.aacn.nche.edu/Media/Factsheets/ImpactEdNp.htm
3. Aiken, L. H., Clarke, S. P., Cheung, R.B., et al. (2003). Educational levels of hospital nurses and surgical patient mortality. *Journal of the American Medical Association, 290,* 1617–1623.

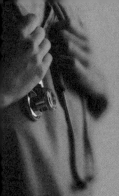

Appendix

TOOLS FOR NURSE LEADERS

CAPITAL EQUIPMENT AQUISITION TOOL

Department _____ Account Number _____ Date: ____
Budgeted Cost _____ Third Party (i.e., MD
Byline, ECRI, etc.) Price Quote Completed __Yes __ No

Name of Equipment:

Equipment Category (Check all that apply.)

___Plant or facilities ___ Separately chargeable to patient

___ Patient care ___ Operating room

___ Safety ___ Software or ___ IS related

___Business/Office ___ Strategic goal related

___ New technology

(1) Will this replace an existing piece of equipment? ___ Yes
___ No

(2) What is the age of equipment being replaced? _____

(3) Has the equipment required increased maintenance? __Yes
___No

   Explain: _____

(4) Will it require a maintenance contract? ___Yes ___No
   If yes, annual cost: _____

(5) Will it require biomedical training and support? __Yes
___No
   If yes, annual cost: ___

(6) Will it require renovation? ___ Yes ___ No
   If yes, annual cost___ and complete renovation request
form.

(7) Will it increase or reduce operating cost? ___ Yes ___ No
   Estimate and type of increase or reduction: _____

(8) Will it increase revenue? ___Yes ___ No

(9) Is it used primarily __ IP or ___ OP
   Yearly Uses: _____ IP yearly uses _____OP yearly
uses

_____
Source: St. Alexius Medical Center Budget Process Worksheet 2008.

Estimate % of use for each patient category_____ IP ____ OP
(10) Will the equipment be used for patients who would constitute an atypical payer mix? (i.e., 99% Medicare, 100% BX BS)

Estimated Payer Mix: _____

(If atypical, you will need to discuss with fiscal to receive
the ROI conversion factors.)

(11) If the item being requested is patient chargeable as
checked above and exceeds $30,000 in cost, complete the
ROI worksheet. If it does not meet the criteria, prepare the
standard capital expenditure request template per policy.

RETURN ON INVESTMENT (ROI) TOOL

Base Cost of Equipment $ _____
Projected Uses/Cases per Year _____:
Inpatient (IP) _____ Outpatient (OP) _____
Useful Life in Years _____
Annual Maintenance Costs _____
Charge per Use: _____
Additional Operating Costs per Year: _____

Net Revenue

Year 1 IP Uses × Charge × 44% IP = Net Year 1 _____
OP Uses 40% OP ———————

Year 2 IP Uses × Charge × 44% IP Net Year 2 _____
OP Uses 40% OP _____

Year 3 IP Uses × Charge × 44% IP = Net Year 3 _____
OP Uses 40% OP _____

Year 4 IP Uses × Charge × 44% IP = Net Year 4 _____
OP Uses 40% OP _____

Year 5 IP Uses × Charge × 44% IP = Net Year 5 _____
OP Uses 40% OP _____

Total Years 1–5 Return = _____

Cost

- Base Cost ÷ Useful Life = Cost/Year
- Renovation Cost ÷ Useful Life = Cost/Year (if applicable)
- Assume 2% of base cost for operating cost unless separately identified:

  Year 1 Cost/Year + Maintenance Cost + Operating Cost (2%)
  Cost Year 1

  Year 2 Cost/Year + Maintenance Cost + Operating Cost (2%) =
  Cost Year 2

  Year 3 Cost/Year + Maintenance Cost + Operating Cost (2%) =
  Cost Year 3

  Year 4 Cost/Year + Maintenance Cost + Operating Cost (2%) =
  Cost Year 4

  Year 5 Cost/Year + Maintenance Cost + Operating Cost (2%) =
  Cost Year 5

  Total Cost Years 1–5 Return =

  Total Net Return 1–5 = ROI

  Total Cost 1–5

Facilities Associated Expense

Renovation: ____No ____Yes (explain):

Electrical Requirements:

Total Renovation Cost:

VENDOR ASSESSMENT TOOL

Vendor	Vendor 1	Vendor 2	Vendor 3
Pros	• Autocharting – no interpretive	• Autocharting – some interpretive	• Auto charting – no interpretive
	• Chalkboard – better than Brand B	• Chalkboard – not as good as Brand A	• Chalkboard – adequate but inferior to Brands A and B
	• Site tailorable	• Site tailorable	• Site tailorable
	• To go live 4 months	• To go live 3–4 months	• Integration with pharmacy
	• Proven track record – 1500 installs nationwide	• Proven track record – 1000 installs nationwide	• Minimal training
	• Bringing up screens – instant	• Bringing up screens – instant unlimited time span viewing for physicians	• Ongoing maintenance and systems administrator could be incorporated in current staff
	• Clinic workstation license available	• Can review chalkboard + strip, full access from Home	• Easy QA
	• Can review chalkboard + strip, configurable from home	• Screen build done	• Unlimited time span view for physicians
	• Screen build done	• Strip review – user determined for time & length	• Integration with medical center
	• Strip review – user determined for time & length	• Annotation boxes on strip more variety to pick from than Brand A	• Screen build done by us – minimal with current Brand Z
	• Annotation boxes on strip more comprehensive, configurable	• Has Labor Curve rated #2 nationally	• Clinic workstation access
	• Has Labor Curve rated #1 nationally		

(Continued)

VENDOR ASSESSMENT TOOL (CONTINUED)

Vendor	Vendor 1	Vendor 2	Vendor 3
Cons	○ Nonintegration with pharmacy (could investigate handheld) ■ 4-hour time span view for physicians ● Requires thick clients, need new PC in every room, more cumbersome » Nonintegration with medical center	○ Nonintegration with pharmacy (could investigate hand held) ● All alarms are charted on strip, including false ● Cannot delete charting that has been charted in error – still shows up » Nonintegration with medical center	■ To go live estimate ?fall, no guarantees on start of installation, need upgrade not slotted until May 1 ▼ No proven track record – 36 installs nationwide ▼ Bringing up screens takes too many seconds, not instant ■ Can review only strip not chalkboard from home currently ■ Strip review – 9 min or 54 min ◆ Annotation boxes on strip more limited ○ No labor curve (questionable could be built in-house) + No national rating
Per Vendor Systems Administrator FTE Support Anticipated	.25 FTE	.25 FTE	.1 FTE
Overall Nursing Score	37.1 (4.6 Average)	27.2 (3.4 Average)	24.7 (3.1 Average)

Source: St. Alexius Medical Center Budget Process Worksheet 2008.

VENDOR SCORES

Scale of 1 – 5 (5 Being Best)

Aggregate Nursing Evaluation Scores	Vendor 1	Vendor 2	Vendor 3
User friendly	4.5	3.3	3
Screens in logical order	4.7	2.6	2.7
Visual layout	4.7	2.6	3.7
Station visibility	4.7	4.3	3.3
Visibility of display in rooms	4.7	3.6	3.3
Pitocin titration	5	3.5	3.0
Ease of charting admission	3.8	3.3	3.7
High-risk charting	5	4	2
Total Nursing Score	37.1 (4.6 Ave)	27.2 (3.4 Ave)	24.7 (3.1 Ave)

Aggregate Nursing Evaluation Scores	Vendor 1	Vendor 2	Vendor 3
Readability of reports	4	3.6	Haven't seen the new ones, Can't determine, current ones Scored 2, 1, NA

Vendor	Vendor 1 Site Visit	Vendor 2 Site Visit	Vendor 3 Live Demo
System Net Price	$326,716.90	$362,489.39	$268,675.00
Service Fee	$195,289.83 (5-Year Term)	$173,266.00 (4-Year Term) 43,316.50 cost/year	$159,020.00 ($31,804 per year)
Labor Curve	NA	NA	$220,000.00 (≈$44,000.00 1 yr × 5 yrs)
Upgrades	NA	NA	$45,000.00 (Approx.)
Thick Clients	$9,900.00	NA	NA
5-Year Comparison	**$531,906.73**	**$579,071.89**	**$692,695.00**

DASHBOARD INDICATORS

Medical Floor–Bed Unit

Indicators	Benchmarks	JULY 2008	AUG 2008	SEPT 2008	OCT 2008	NOV 2008
Financial Indicators						
Expenses %	budget	−.50	2.84	15.39	2.9	5.06
Revenue %	budget	−8.43	3.06	2.99	2.46	6.80
Total Worked HPPD [Direct/Indirect]	9.22-9.80 9.51	9.21	8.95	8.53	8.54	8.78
Total Paid HPPD	11.10	11.02	10.20	10.49	10.17	10.24
Volume Indicators						
Total Patient Days # of Admits	782.5	807	863	836	842	837
IP	144.7	145	166	140	147	139
24-Hour Holds	83.7	144	111	91	61	94
ADC	25.73	26.03	27.84	27.87	27.16	27.9
ALOS	4.83-3.43	4.5 2.79	4.53 3.12	5.32 3.62	5.31 4.05	5.35 3.59
Customer Service Indicators						
Patient Opinion Survey	84-89			82.7		
Human Resource Indicators						
Sick Time [Hrs & %]	<3%	298 3.87%	210 2.74	327.5 4.01	304.75 3.83	738.75 6.30
Incentive $		100 788	300 459 484	860 550	200 0	0 366
Overtime [Hrs & %]	<2%	58.5 .76%	89.75 1.17	117.25 1.44	104 1.31	92.25 .78

DEC 2008	JAN 2009	FEB 2009	MAR 2009	APRIL 2009	MAY 2009	JUNE 2009	YTD
3.84	7.02	2.71	4.58	6.55	6.13	16.29	6.07
−1.22	−3.70	−.05	3.84	4.81	3.73	2.34	1.39
9.08	8.94	9.02	8.75	8.77	9.0	8.71	8.86
11.09	10.79	10.06	10.05	9.84	10.21	10.82	10.42
805	828	772	851	849	822	813	827
134	136	133	150	142	142	120	141
80	77	78	111	76	114	113	96
25.97	26.71	27.57	27.45	28.3	26.52	27.10	27.20
5.41 3.76	5.52 3.89	5.22 3.66	4.93 3.26	5.44 3.89	4.99 3.21	5.83 3.49	5.20 3.53
84.7			83.9			83.7	
405.75 5.12	309.75 3.91	157 1.97	66.5 .88	937 4.97	293 2.52	179.25 2.13	307 3.51
390 16	250 650 500	100 0	300 150	374 116	100 150	458 500	8,161
64 .81	76.5 .97	50 .63	47.75 .63	84.5 1.07	78 .67	113.5 1.35	81.3 .97

Indicators	Benchmarks	JULY 2009	AUG 2009	SEPT 2009	OCT 2009	NOV 2009
Staffing Efficiency RN/ Extender	4SW 4SC	Not Avail	Not Avail	Not Avail	Not Avail	Not Avail
**Turnover Total RN LPN						
Open Positions/ Detail [FTE's]	Detail 25.04 RN 1.22 RN Flex 8.4 LPN 7.0 NA 1.34 NA Flex 4.9 CC	.46 −.62 −1.40 −1.5 .05 −.60	.28 .28 −1.4 −2.2 .06 −.60	−.54 .28 −.50 −2.5 .06 −.10	-.73 .28 .40 -2.6 .05 -.10	.16 .28 −.40 −1.60 .05 −.10
Quality Indicators						
Total # of Falls		6	5	6	3	5
Total Med Errors		8	5	7	6	1
Pressure Ulcers		0	0	1	0	0
Barcoding %	90% 4SC 4SW	90.88 94.64	93 94.7	91.9 92.2	93.35 93.48	90.6 89.6
Advance Directives	90% 4SC 4SW	88% 95%			86 100	
Code Level	4SC 4SW	50% 100%			100 100	
Call Light # calls/ response time	4SC 4SW	4423 1:33 3351 1:19	4756 1:30 3417 1:34	5315 1:35 3581 1:41	5086 1:36 3475 1:29	4365 1:39 3705 1:32
Hospital Acquired Infections		2	1	1	1	3

This dashboard is an example of the type of form that could be placed on unit staff bulletin boards, shared at unit meetings and used for annual staff leadership job performance appraisals.

DEC 2009	JAN 2010	FEB 2010	MAR 2010	APRIL 2010	MAY 2010	JUNE 2010	YTD
Not Avail	Not Avail	Not Avail	Not Avail	Not Avail	Not Avail	Not Avail	Not Avail
−.24 .28 −1.4 −1.6 .05 −1.0	.26 −.62 −.5 −.20 .05 −.10	−.24 −.62 −.50 −.90 .05 −.20	0 −.62 −.50 0 .05 −.20	0 −.62 −.50 −1.3 .05 −.20	.96 −.62 −.50 −.80 .05 .30	.96 −.62 −1.4 −.40 .05 −.20	
6	2	3	5	5	5	5	56
1	10	10	5	1	6	4	64
0	0	0	0	0	0	0	1
93.3 93.3	92.2 94.1	92.6 93.7	91.49 94.82	92.1 94.3	93.8 94.1	92.15 93.62	
	88 91			100 100			97 95
	83 100			100 78			78 100
5305 1:23 3639 1:23	4196 1:22 3463 1:28	4973 1:23 2891 1:12	5358 1:3 4048 1:10	4777 1:23 4595 1:36	5183 1:35 3964 1:40	5656 1:27 3369 1:50	
4	3	3	0	1	1		20

MEDICAL/ONCOLOGY SCOPE/ PLAN OF CARE 2008–2009

Unit Description

The medical/oncology unit is a 31-bed inpatient unit. 4th floor, south center nurses station (4SC)—17 beds consist of medical patients; and 4th floor south west nurses station (4SW)—14 beds consist of oncology patients, hospice-allocated rooms, and medical overflow. In addition to providing care to the medical/oncology patients, the unit also provides the capability of remote cardiac monitoring. The Stroke Center is located on 4SC with allocated rooms. The JCAHO-certified Stroke Center has been created to improve the overall quality of care for people afflicted by stroke.

Population and Type of Patients Served

The predominant patient populations served are adult and geriatric patients. An occasional adolescent patient may be admitted to the unit. The predominant diagnostic group served is adult medical and oncology patients.

Criteria for Entry, Admission, and Treatment

Patients are admitted to the department based on established admission criteria. The credentialed physician makes arrangements for admission.

Frequent Procedures/Services/Process

The care is provided through a multidisciplinary team approach. The most frequent patient populations are: diabetic, cerebrovascular accident, nutritional/metabolic, infectious disease, cardiorespiratory, cancer-related, chemotherapy, hospice patients, and other medical complications in adult care. Family and significant other support is provided by nursing staff in collaboration with the other multidisciplinary team members. All cancer patients admitted to the oncology unit have an automatic multidisciplinary screening criteria completed.

Hours and Days of Operation

The medical/oncology unit is open 24 hours a day, 7 days a week.

The budgeted average daily census is 27.

The oncology census is supplemented with overflow patients who are noninfectious or have a nonviral diagnosis.

The medical/oncology unit is budgeted for 9.22–9.80 (average 9.51) productive hours per patient day and 11.10 paid hours per patient day.

Service Delivery Sites

Functional therapies are provided in respective departments.

Assessment of Patient Needs and Treatment

Evaluation/assessment is performed by a registered nurse. Assessment includes review of medical records, patient (or responsible guardian) interview, physical and functional assessment. Based on the assessment, a plan of care is established and implemented. The patient and/or authorized guardian is involved in the plan of care and related goals. Treatment is offered through our multidisciplinary continuance of care.

Support Services Provided by Hospital and Referral Contacts

Medical support is available during all hours of department operation through the emergency department, hospitalists, intensivists, and physician call schedules. Facilities support (environmental services, maintenance, etc.) is also available during all hours of department operation through direct contact with facilities support departments or via beeper. Systems support (information systems, central supply, etc.) is also available during all hours of operation through direct contact with system support departments or via beeper.

Scope of Service

The medical/oncology unit's primary customers are the patients and their families. Internally, the medical oncology customers are defined as those departments that interact with the medical/oncology unit. A comprehensive list of internal customers would be lengthy, but some examples include:

- Other nursing units pertaining to patient care functions
- Health information services pertaining to current/prior patient medical records
- Pharmacy pertaining to patient medications and education
- Laboratory and radiology for patient diagnostic testing and data
- Anesthesiology pertaining to patient care
- Admitting pertaining to patient demographics and admission and discharge
- Respiratory, physical, occupational, and speech therapy pertaining to patient care
- Social services pertaining to discharge planning and other patient needs
- Quality management pertaining to utilization review

External customers include:

- Physicians and their office personnel
- Referring physicians and their office personnel
- Other health care institutions

Nursing Delivery Model

The Patient Care Team is the patient care delivery model utilized at St. Alexius. This model was developed uniquely by the medical center staff and leadership in response to the rapid and continuous changes in health care, and the unique needs of each nursing unit and their patient populations. The nursing delivery model, Patient Care Team, is a unique model of care which is provided on the medical/oncology unit and at St. Alexius that supports a team approach to effectively and efficiently meet the needs of our patients and their families. Each unit is specialized in serving different patient populations with unique needs, therefore operationalization of the model may vary between units. The team of staff may vary on each unit as well. Consistent with the state Nurse Practice Act and the state's Board of Nursing Administrative Rules. The common element required on each unit is that the registered nurse (RN) will be responsible and accountable for the delivery of patient care, the licensed practical nurse (LPN) works under the direction of the RN and assists in implementing the nursing process, and the unlicensed assistive personnel (UAP) work under the direction of a licensed nurse. The ANA Code of Ethics for Nurses and the RN Bill of Rights are integrated into practice at all levels of the nursing organization.

Department Organizational Structure

The director of the medical/oncology unit is responsible for the organization, planning, and daily operation of the unit. The director reports to the senior vice president/chief nursing officer.

The clinical coordinator of the medical/oncology unit is responsible for assessing, planning, implementing, evaluating, and supervising unit activities according to unit policies and procedures while maintaining standards of nursing practice. The clinical coordinator remains clinically competent in the event patient care needs require assistance and at least 36 hours per month he or she is assigned shifts on the unit to assure the necessary unit-based competencies. The clinical coordinator reports to the director of the medical/oncology unit.

The Medical Centers' Division of Nursing uses a Shared Governance professional practice model that is based on a foundation of decentralized decision making. The Shared Governance model is built on a structure that supports the point-of-care provider and sustains ownership and accountability to improve and provide safe patient care.

Staffing Plan

The Division of Nursing utilizes the American Nurses Association Nurse Staffing Standards, the Medical Center Staffing Scheduling Standard Operating Procedure, and unit-specific policies and procedures to guide staffing decisions. In the determination of appropriate staffing, the Division of Nursing evaluates, on a continuous basis, unit functions necessary to support the delivery of quality patient care, patient-based needs, the aggregate population of patients, and the associated roles and responsibilities of the nursing staff. These include, but are not limited to:

- Number of patients/patient acuity/medications provided
- Levels of intensity of the patients for whom care is being provided
- Architecture and geography of the environment
- Available technology
- Patient outcome information that focuses on Continuous Quality Improvement (CQI) issues
- Level of preparation/experience/competency of providers.

Productivity is monitored to reflect efficient use of staffing resources. Patient outcome data is utilized to measure the effectiveness of resource allocations.

The current staffing plan is based upon current workload of 9.51 budgeted productive nursing hours per patient day with an average daily census of 27 patients. Staffing patterns are evaluated three times per day through the analysis of patient volumes, patient acuity, and nurse-to-patient ratios. The master staffing plan is variable, based on the daily staffing guidelines. Staffing variances are handled by:

- Calling in additional staff members
- Reassigning qualified staff members from another unit
- Prioritizing and reassigning duties when workload exceeds staffing levels
- Reassigning personnel to another unit where needed
- Giving personal or a low census day off

The medical/oncology unit is staffed with RNs, LPNs, VAPs Practical Nurses, and communication clerks.

Medical/Oncology Staffing

Hours Per Patient Day

Productive: 9.22–9.88 (average: 9.51)

Paid: 11.10

%Care/Shift	Direct Care RN/LPN/UAP	
Days: 41%	RN 4 / LPN 4 / UAP 3	HPPD: 3.47
Eves: 37%	RN 4 / LPN 4 / NA 2	HPPD: 2.96
Nocs: 22.2%	RN 4 / LPN 1 / NA 0	HPPD: 1.78

Total FTEs	Skill Mix
Director: .34	RN – 62%
Asst. Director: 1.00	LPN – 21%
Team Leader: 1.00	NA – 17%
RN: 24.40	
RN Flex Pool 1.22	
LPN 8.40	
NA 7.00	
NA Flex Pool 1.34	
Clerk 4.90	

Total: 49.14

Vacation Assignment

Vacations are granted based on patient care needs. As a general rule, 1–2 vacation/leave requests per RN, LPN, and nurse assistant are granted at one time on the day and evening shift, and one nurse on the night shift. Additional vacation may be granted with short notice.

Emergency Plan

In the event of a severe emergency such as a severe weather condition or a disaster, the minimum amount of staff required to safely operate this unit with a 89% occupancy or less is based on acuity with an average of 27 patients. This is combining the medical and oncology units.

- Day shift: 2 RN, 1 LPN, 1 NA
- Eve shift: 2 RN, 1 LPN, 1 NA
- Night Shift: 2 RN, 1 LPN

Staff Qualifications

Team Leader

The basic requirements for team leader include:
- Current North Dakota licensure
- Current basic life support (BLS) card
- Satisfactory completion of competency-based orientation (CBO) program
- Must to be nationally certified within 1 year

Registered Nurse

The basic requirements for RN staff include:
- Current North Dakota licensure
- Current BLS card
- Satisfactory completion of CBO program

Licensed Practical Nurse

The basic requirements for LPN staff include:
- Current North Dakota licensure
- Current BLS card
- IV Therapy Certification
- Satisfactory completion of CBO program

Unlicensed Assistive Personnel

The basic requirements for UAP staff include:
- Current North Dakota Registry card
- Current BLS card
- Satisfactory completion of CBO program

Communication Clerks

The basic requirements for communication clerks include:
- Current BLS card
- Typing and clerical skills
- Satisfactory completion of CBO program

Unit Education Plan

An education plan is developed annually to meet the needs of the medical/oncology unit. This plan is based on a needs assessment completed by the staff, new technology, medications, high risk/low volume, procedures being utilized in the departments, quality review findings, changes in patient population, etc. Education is provided at in-service and/or meetings and the staff is encouraged to attend appropriate outside conferences or in-service trainings. In addition to this education, staff participates in hospitalwide safety, infection control, electrical safety, life support education. Record of in-service topics and attendance are kept in the Education Department. (See attached Education Plan)

Orientation

Staff on the medical/oncology unit participates in the appropriate hospital orientation programs. Unit orientation follows a Competency-Based Orientation model, with a preceptor assigned to the employee until he or she has completed the level of orientation that allows him or her to function independently. Orientation records are maintained in the human resources department.

Ongoing Competency Evaluation

Validation of selected skills occurs annually in the department. Skill competency to be evaluated is determined based on patient care needs, new technology, new procedures, high-risk or low-volume skills, quality review findings, changes in patient population, new medications, etc. Annual job performance appraisals validate competency in general.

Job Performance Appraisal

Job performance appraisals are performed in accordance with the St. Alexius human resource policies.

Department leadership is evaluated annually by the senior vice president/chief nursing officer, staff representatives, physician representatives, and key customers of the medical/ oncology unit.

Customer satisfaction is evaluated through the patient opinion survey process. Job performance standards are reviewed and revised on an annual basis.

Policies and Procedures

The medical/oncology unit follows the general administrative Division of Nursing policies and procedures.

New policies and procedures are developed as needed for new equipment, procedures, etc., when introduced in the department. Resources used to develop the policies are standards of practice and care, manufacturer information, and physician, nursing, or other professional input.

Policies are reviewed at a minimum of every 3 years. New and revised policies require input of clinical nursing staff and other multidisciplinary units as required along with administrative approval prior to implementation. In-service education of the policy and procedure is provided through memos, staff meetings, skilled labs, or through an educational in-service training.

Standards of Practice/Standards of Care/Performance Improvement

The medical/oncology unit utilizes JCAHO standards, the state Nurse Practice Act, the American Nurses Association Scope and Standards of Clinical Nursing Practice, and *Patient Care Standards*, by Susan Marie Tucker et al. (7th ed., Mosby, 2000) as resources in the development of policies and procedures.

Standards of care are based on an interdisciplinary delivery model and relate to assessment, planning of patient care, physical and psychosocial needs, discharge planning, and patient and family education. These standards are available in the departmental policy and procedure manual.

Performance Improvement

The medical/oncology unit staff share the overall mission, vision, and values of the Medical Center. They are committed to providing expert, compassionate care to all individuals who present to the medical/oncology unit and to the family members who provide support to them.

The medical/oncology unit participates in the Quality Improvement Program of the Medical Center. A department quality committee meets monthly or as needed. Reports are presented to staff via written and verbal communication channels.

The medical/oncology unit participates in the Quality Improvement Program of the Medical Center. A department nursing care council committee meets monthly or as needed. Reports are presented to the staff via written and verbal communication channels.

The medical/oncology unit is involved in the following performance improvement activities and monitors:

- Pain monitor
- Braden Risk Assessment Scale
- Restraints
- Crash cart/defibrillator checks
- Fall risk assessment
- Patient education monitor
- Code status monitor
- Patient opinion survey
- Preinvasive procedure verification
- Mission effectiveness projects
- Medication refrigerator temperatures

Data related to the following nurse-sensitive indicators are collected at the unit level:

- Maintenance of skin integrity; pressure ulcer prevalence and occurrence
- Nursing hours provided per patient day (HPPD)
- Nursing satisfaction

- Patient injury rates (falls)
- Patient satisfaction in relation to nursing care, pain management, patient education, and overall care.
- Skill mix of RNs, LPNs, and unlicensed staff.

A number of units participate in the National Database for Nursing Quality Indicators (NDNQI), which provides national benchmarking opportunities.

In addition, the medical/oncology unit collects data on the following nurse-sensitive quality indicators: medication errors, hospital-acquired infections, and patient falls. These indicators are collected at the unit level, trended over time, and analyzed for impact on patient outcomes.

The indicators are trended on the unit dashboards. Outcomes may be reported in annual reports, annual reviews of the performance improvement plan, and/or at staff meetings.

Another analysis that occurs on a monthly basis is to review two human resource indicators and two clinical indicators for staffing effectiveness. For the medical/oncology unit, the indicators are HPPD, turnover, medication errors, and falls. These indicators are reviewed in relationship to each other and visualized on control charts. Any occurrences outside of the range of expected performance requires a report of actions to the staffing effectiveness committee.

Performance improvement activities are analyzed and reported on a quarterly basis, and action is taken as appropriate. An annual review of activities is performed and adjustments are made by the staff representatives on the quality improvement committee, with input from the director and the assistant director. Results are reported at staff meetings and monitors being conducted are reviewed with the staff.

Goal Setting

Unit goals are developed by unit staff and management on an annual basis. Responsibility for developing and carrying forward a plan to meet those goals in assigned to staff representatives. Updates are completed and presented to staff, management, and administration on a quarterly basis. Each staff member is required to actively participate in meeting the goals, and a percentage of each individual's performance appraisal is dependent on successful completion of those goals. Individuals also set professional goals for themselves as part of their performance appraisal.

The 2008–2009 medical/oncology department goals are: Develop and implement formalized strategies to address age-related diagnostic and therapeutic modalities and programs that ensure St. Alexius Medical Center is on the "cutting edge" of quality service delivery in oncology.

Ongoing Assessment of Resources

Financial review is conducted on a monthly basis, with comparison of actual revenue and expense, volume, and productivity standards to budgeted numbers. At a minimum of annually, this information is used to predict needs for the upcoming fiscal year. The director, staff, and physicians provide input on capital equipment needs and any potential for development of new services. Departmental and hospital activity are reported periodically through written and verbal communication channels. The budget for the upcoming year is reviewed with staff after board approval.

Communication/Collaboration/Functional Relationships with Other Departments and Services

Communication Methodology

Internal communications are organized around monthly staff meetings and unit nursing practice council meetings. A communication book is maintained in the department. Memos, letters, notes, etc., are placed in the communication book. All staff members are responsible for reading the communication book on a regular basis. Voice mail or e-mail may also be used to communicate.

External communications occur between referring physicians, their clinic staff, and other health care providers via telephone, e-mail, regular mail, or scheduled meetings as necessary.

Collaborative and Functional Relationships

The medical/oncology unit recognizes that clinical care is a collaborative effort with other professions and other departments. Medical/oncology unit staff interact with colleagues of other nursing units such as the intensive care unit (ICU), telemetry, transitional care unit (TCU), rehab, and surgical unit. Such interaction may involve nursing consultations, referrals for additional services, transfers of patient care, etc. Interaction also occurs with other disciplines, such as physical therapy, occupational therapy, respiratory care, social services, pastoral care, dietary, pharmacy, etc., for patient care planning, patient and family education, and discharge planning. Representatives of other disciplines serve on process improvement teams and participate in staff meetings as appropriate.

Medical/oncology unit staff collaborate with clinical and non-clinical areas to facilitate smooth, seamless patient flow through the continuum of care for the persons served through the department.

Developed:	93
Reviewed/revised:	94-02, 03, 11/04, 06/05, 03/06, 05/06, 05/07, 04/08
Dept. responsible:	Medical
Resource:	Unit director

Source: St. Alexius Medical Center Plan for the Provision of Care 2008.

QUALITY AND SAFETY MONITORING FACESHEET

Title: _____ Date Developed: _____

Describe the objective of the monitor:

Describe expected improvements:

List the indicators to be monitored:

1.

2.

3.

Describe the methodology to be used for the data collection, i.e., sampling, 100% review: How frequently will the data be collected? What time frame will be used to collect the data?

Where will the findings be reported: _____

Date findings will be reported: _____

Responsible party signature _____ Date :_____

QUALITY AND SAFETY MONITORING EVALUATION FORM

Department:_____ Date Reported: _____

Monitor Title: _____ Time Frame Studied: _____

List Indicators: List Benchmark:

1.

2.

3.

Findings:

Analysis:

Action plan based on findings and analysis:

Signature of individual completing report:_____
_____Date:____

QUALITY AND SAFETY MONITORING TREND FORM

DEPARTMENT: _____

Indicators	Benchmark	JAN	FEB	MAR	APR	MAY	JUN	JUL	AUG	SEP	OCT	NOV	DEC

Source: St. Alexius Medical Center Quality Plan and Program.

Index

Page numbers followed by italic *f* and *t* indicate figures and tables, respectively.